# Extraordinary Women in Science & Medicine:
# Four Centuries of Achievement

AN EXHIBITION AT THE GROLIER CLUB, NEW YORK

18 SEPTEMBER – 23 NOVEMBER 2013

# EXTRAORDINARY WOMEN IN SCIENCE & MEDICINE

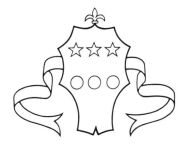

# Four Centuries of Achievement

Ronald K. Smeltzer

Robert J. Ruben

Paulette Rose

## The Grolier Club

New York · 2013

ISBN 978-1-60583-047-x

# TABLE OF CONTENTS

# PREFACE

## INTRODUCTION

This Grolier Club exhibition, "Extraordinary Women in Science and Medicine: Four Centuries of Achievement," focuses on the history and outstanding achievements of women in the sciences. Within the educational and professional communities, women's participation in the sciences continues as a major topic of discussion and concern. Their entry and success in the physical and medical sciences, engineering, and mathematics vary widely among subject areas. In the medical sciences, women now constitute almost fifty percent of new students, but women in leadership positions are few. In most other fields, women continue to make at best modest, incremental advances. Remarkably, in computer science, fewer women than ever are involved in the scientific and technical communities.

The exhibition and its catalog are designed to engage the visitor by revealing the human stories behind the careers and accomplishments of thirty-two exceptional women in science since the seventeenth century. Of the women included here, most are well known within the scientific community but very few have broad recognition. Our intention is to raise awareness and understanding of women's roles in the development of the sciences by chronicling, with primary source documents, their major contributions in science and technology.

In presenting the brief biographies of the women, the curators have tried, in particular, to capture the aspects of their lives that seemed to be significant in the development of their scientific careers and to highlight the factors that contributed to their success and recognition – or lack thereof. For example, the often-proscribed educational opportunities available to the women are noted, and how our subjects overcame limitations imposed by contemporary society and the academy are examined. In some cases, the availability of role models was important. Gender discrimination, sometimes on an individual basis and sometimes organizational and societal, is a recurring theme. The exhibition and this catalog may suggest many questions to elucidate how women have fared in the scientific community since the early seventeenth century.

Among the questions that the exhibition invites viewers to consider are the following: How important for recognition were the limited educational opportunities, and how did some women overcome the lack of a formal education? How significant were role models and mentors? How effective were women in the use of social capital and in participation in scientific networks? Did individual styles of doing science – analytical, model building, data-intensive, and intuitive – affect outcomes? How did different types of achievement – significant discoveries versus, for example, development of experimental methods, intense data gathering, and proving theories proposed by others – affect recognition? Is observation without interpretation discovery? How was gender discrimination manifested? Were gender issues considered significant by the women themselves? What role did marriage and family play in their careers? And how important was the role of finding the right mentor in their scientific careers? These questions are relevant in different ways for the accomplishments of the thirty-two women singled out in this exhibition. The viewers are invited to consider these questions as they ponder who did and who did not receive recognition – for example Nobel awards among the modern women researchers and general historical acknowledgment among the women from earlier eras.

## SCOPE AND ORGANIZATION

For the time frame, the curators decided to consider the period after scientific studies broke free from the concept of ancient authority as the source of knowledge, thus suggesting the seventeenth century as the earliest period from which to identify women who were significant figures in the sciences. Consequently, the earliest women included are a practitioner of obstetrics and gynecology who became midwife to King Henry IV and Catherine de Medici of France and a remarkable Polish author on mathematical astronomy, writing while in refuge from the horror of the Thirty Years' War.

Looking ahead from the seventeenth century and taking into account the spectacular development of science during the twentieth century, two time periods with different criteria for the selection of the women were adopted as an organizing principle. For the period before the mid-nineteenth century, women with significant discoveries to their name are few. Therefore, for this early period, the criterion adopted was to consider women with published works that at the very least created an innovative and important synthesis of state-of-the-art knowledge. From the mid-nineteenth century onward, the primary criterion adopted was that published work must be associated with significant discoveries that represent important new knowledge. No women still living are included.

A preliminary list of women the curators considered eligible for inclusion was winnowed by a number of factors. First, there had to be pertinent material available to exhibit for everyone chosen. This factor turned out to be significant in the medical sciences, as the proposal to include Maria Dalle Donne and Anna Morandi Manzolini could not be supported by the availability of exhibition material. A number of women who authored scientific texts were excluded because their work seemed purely secondary in nature. In some cases, the women seemed to have been adjuncts rather than original contributors. In other cases, their work seemed to be purely didactic. Ultimately, of course, the women and the materials had to be identified to fit the exhibition space.

The scope of the exhibition is organized generally by technical subjects within two major groupings: the physical sciences and the medical sciences. Outside the scope of the exhibition is natural history, which the curators view as a unique subject of its own.

To represent the physical sciences, the curators selected twenty-three women. Their work is organized among five subject areas: physics, chemistry, astronomy, mathematics, and computing. One question of terminology that requires clarification is that what today is called physics was earlier called "natural philosophy" or a similar term. For the most part, it was a straightforward task to situate the scientists within the five subject fields. Physics is the largest category, with nine representatives: two from the eighteenth century and seven from the twentieth century. The Curies, Marie and her daughter Irène, were considered appropriate for the physics, not chemistry, category, because their work and discoveries were more relevant to the development of nuclear and particle physics than to topics in chemistry. The other subject areas, with the exception of computing, have representatives that span more than three and a half centuries of scientific work.

Nine women active in the medical sciences from the early seventeenth century until the middle of the twentieth century are included. Three of these added to fundamental medical knowledge in obstetrics, women's health, and cardiology; three worked in genetics and cell biology; and three worked in biochemistry. Each overcame barriers based upon gender issues, adapting in one way or another to obstacles. Each pursued her path to discovery, which resulted, in all cases in substantial gains for all of humanity. The world is a healthier and better place for their contributions, and much of current medical science is based upon their discoveries.

The exhibition contains a wide variety of types of publications, some of which are not generally seen in non-scientific fields, but are very significant in the sciences. In addition to periodicals and monographs, important scientific discoveries can be found in dissertations and theses, the proceedings of conferences, published lectures, reports issued by institutions, formerly classified documents, and various types of manuscript materials, perhaps never published. An important type of publication in the sciences is authors' separates, which can be preprints, offprints, and reprints of serial or conference papers. The significance of authors' separates can vary greatly, depending upon their relationship in time to the formal publication of the work in a more widely circulated form. For the modern period of this exhibition, the majority of scientific discoveries became generally known from serial publications, not from later circulation of authors' offprints. Especially for the modern period, the exhibition includes many examples of the less common types of scientific publications.

Publications and objects with special attributes and interesting features are found throughout the exhibition. The opportunity is taken to announce the discovery of the false attribution of first edition to a seventeenth-century book: examination of the book revealed what must be a previously unnoticed, typesetting error in the date on the title page (cat. no. 87). A remarkable survivor in an eighteenth-century book is a leaf that was excised and replaced by a new leaf, because the author changed her mind about the text; the excised leaf, preserved with the book, allows the reader to know the author's original thoughts (cat. no. 8). One of the most important breakthroughs in modern genetics is first recorded, uniquely, on a brown paper bag (cat. no. 147). Uncommon and interesting aspects of printing are illustrated by such items as a book printed in the typeface, *Roman du Roi*, commissioned by King Louis XIV for the Imprimerie Royale (cat. no. 6); early books showing the typesetting of mathematical equations (cat. no. 68); and books with early technical and decorative engravings (cat. nos. 4 and 9). A number of publications have interesting associations, and one book is from the library of Talleyrand with his bookplate (cat. no. 13).

Turning to the catalog, the reader is encouraged to focus on two preceding essays by invited academics, presenting an overview of the history and future of women in science. Each of the curators' essays begins with a concise scientific biography, emphasizing how gender issues influenced career paths and recognition. Following each biography is a brief summary describing the significance of the subject's accomplishments. Both of these sections are documented by endnotes with citations to the subject's publications and to scholarly articles about her work. A major effort was made to describe the women's achievements without the use of undefined scientific jargon – not an easy task in some cases when discussing theoretical physics and mathematics. Provided also is a suggested reading list for each woman. The final section of each essay describes the items in the exhibition. Many are milestone publications, serving in some cases to supplement the important publications listed in the endnotes. Notable items in the exhibition include a piece of scientific hardware used by Marie Curie (cat. no. 27). Also included are a few items that emphasize aspects of the human story of the women beyond their scientific work.

## A NOTE TO THE READER

Two general rules for the spelling of the women's names were adopted. In the texts, the modern, standard spelling is used for names. In citations to original publications, the names of the women are preserved with the original spelling, presumably as the author wanted her name spelled at the time. In one case, the woman's choices about the use of her married name can be tracked over time. In general, the spellings in older publications are preserved. In French, all spellings are preserved. For example, the title of Voltaire's book on Newton has spellings *Elémens* and *Neuton.*

Authors of the biographical essays are identified by initials. In addition to the curators, other authors are Yvonne Korshak, Ph.D. (YK) and P. J. Mode (PJM).

ACKNOWLEDGMENTS

The rare and unusual publications and objects in this exhibition have been generously loaned by private individuals and institutions. The curators deeply appreciate the loans. The exhibition labels identify the lenders who wish to be recognized.

For the institutional loans, the curators express their appreciation for the help and courtesies of the following individuals. At the Chemical Heritage Foundation, James Voelkel, curator of rare books, Othmer Library of Chemical History, facilitated our requests and was kind enough to provide answers to research queries. At Bryn Mawr College, Eric L. Pumroy, director of Library Collections, and Seymour Adelman, head of Special Collections, kindly allowed us to select our choice of items. The efforts of Jennifer B. Lee, curator for Performing Arts, Rare Book and Manuscript Library, Columbia University, to assist in the loan selection process were essential; also at Columbia University, the support of Michael T. Ryan, director of the Rare Book and Manuscript Library was likewise vital. At The Huntington Library, Daniel Lewis, Dibner senior curator, History of Science and Technology and chief curator of manuscripts, opened the path for a loan request.

Additional institutional loans were organized by Arlene Shaner, acting curator of the Rare Books and Manuscripts Library of the New York Academy of Medicine; in addition to kindly permitting the use of several items from the collection of this institution, she provided superb advice and identified heretofore unappreciated works. One key item in the exhibition was arranged through the courtesy of Bruce Bradley, librarian for History of Science, and Lisa Browar, president of the Linda Hall Library. At the University of Chicago Library, Daniel Meyer, director of the Special Collections Research Center, kindly supported a request for a rare volume. Chris Petersen, faculty research assistant and specialist for the Linus Pauling Archive at the Special Collections and Archives Research Center, Oregon State University, assisted in the selection of one loan item. At the College of Physicians of Philadelphia, Robert D. Hicks, director, Mutter Museum and Historical Library, and Anna Dhody, curator, Mutter Museum, were instrumental for the loan of a large piece of scientific apparatus. In addition to arranging a loan, John E. Mustain, Special Collections librarian, Cecil H. Green Library, Stanford University provided a key item of information from a book in the collection.

Further institutional loans originated with Melissa Grafe and Florence Gillich at the John R. Bumstead Library for Medical History, Cushing/Whitney Medical Library of Yale University, who graciously provided both a loan and an image of a very rare item. The National Library of Medicine, through the good offices of Michael J. North and Stephen J. Greenberg, facilitated the loan of three items with images and a complete scan of two of them. Phoebe Evans Letocha and Andrew Harrison at the Alan Mason Chesney Medical Archives, Johns Hopkins Medical Institutions helped in every way possible in providing access to their extensive archives, and enabling a loan and two images of primary data. The American Philosophical Society provided an ideal environment for accessing archives, as well as the much-appreciated knowledgeable advice of Charles Greifenstein, and loans of images that were expedited by Valerie-Ann Lutz. Barbara R. Tysinger at the Health Sciences Library, University of North Carolina at Chapel Hill kindly provided the loan of a key item. At the Cold Spring Harbor Laboratory Archives, Clare Clark and Ludmila Pollock gave generously of their time and deep knowledge of their collection in aiding the selection of material for the exhibition. Professor Phillippe Lefebrve of the University of Liège and Aldo Cicinelli in the Secretariat of the Pontificia Accademia delle Scienze each generously provided copies of critical publications.

Loans are gratefully acknowledged from private collections. Ellen Heffelfinger, librarian for the Fry's Electronics Collection, was gracious in offering a long list of items from this private collection. Professor Gerald L. Alexanderson, Santa Clara University, graciously agreed to lend items from his collection. P. J. Mode, fellow Grolier Club member, kindly lent one item. Colin Franklin graciously allowed us to use an interesting personal letter. We were able to include a very special object in the exhibition through the courtesy of Jenny P. Glusker. Dr. Jon Elion sought out and has loaned one very poignant manuscript. Otherwise, the remaining unidentified materials are from the collections of the three curators, Ronald K. Smeltzer, Robert J. Ruben, and Paulette Rose.

In addition to the loan of items included in the exhibition, thanks are due for many other reasons. Portraits and images provided gratuitously originated with Mikael Rågstedt, librarian, Institut Mittag-Leffler; Marta Cavazza, professor, University of Bologna, Archivio di Stato di Bologna; Dr. Radoslaw Skowron, Museum Dawnego Kupiectwa Úwidnicy; Maria Rentetzi, professor, National Technical University of Athens; Artur Svansson; and Keith R. Fletcher for the firms of H. M. Fletcher and Nigel Phillips. We want to thank Sharon Bertsch McGrayne, writer and scholar, for her personal contribution of significant material accompanied by sage advice.

For research assistance and suggestions, acknowledgments are due to Elizabeth Crawford, Peggy Kidwell, Alison Doane, Grazyna Meray, and Arnold Perlmutter.

William Tobin kindly undertook a research task that provided important information. Robert Lorenzson, a master photographer, made the photographs for many of our catalog illustrations. Robert J. Ruben wishes to specially acknowledge his longtime editing and writing collaborator, his wife Yvonne Ruben, professional name Yvonne Korshak.

Members and staff of The Grolier Club whose assistance has been especially important are: Director Eric J. Holzenberg; Exhibitions Coordinator Megan Smith; and George Ong, chair of the Committee on Publications. For help at critical times we especially thank fellow Grolier Club members Jane Randall and Kathryn Rodgers. We extend our appreciation to Susan Flamm for her invaluable assistance in bringing the exhibition to the attention of the public at large. Finally, the vision, design talent and production expertise of Jerry Kelly were essential to the production of the catalog.

The exhibition and its catalog were made possible by the generous participation of many organizations and individuals. Very special thanks for a generous grant are due The Gladys Krieble Delmas Foundation; Deirdre C. Stam and David Stam were essential to this assistance. A generous grant from The Arthur F. & Alice E. Adams Charitable Foundation is especially acknowledged; we are indebted to Arete Warren for her help to make this happen. Businesses due very special thanks are Libreria Antiquaria Mediolanum, Herman H. J. Lynge & Son, Sophia Rare Books, and Deborah Coltham Rare Books. We thank Linda Brodsky, M.D. for her deep sympathy with our goals and her significant assistance.

We are deeply grateful to a number of dear friends and colleagues who responded generously to the purposes and meaning of our exhibition, including Gerald L. Alexanderson, Joan and Peter Arvedson, Ph.D., Linda Brodsky, M.D. and Saul Greenfield, M.D., Linda M. Miller Calandra, RN, Robin T. Cotton, M.D., Craig S. Derkay, M.D., Adele Evans, Sanford E. Gerber, Ph.D., Arielle Kauvar, M.D., Joyce Lowinson, M.D., Julie Mitnick, M.D., Maureen E. Mulvihill, Ph.D., Jennifer Schloss, Richard Schwartz, M.D., Tania Sih, M.D., Steven Sobol, M.D., Cynthia Solot and Steven Handler, M.D., Dana M. Thompson, M.D., Debra G. Weinberger, M.D., Ralph Wetmore, M.D., and Brian J. and Deborah W. Wiatrak, M.D.

Finally, the curators wish to acknowledge and extend their appreciation to Joseph M. Rose and Suzanne C. Smeltzer for their enthusiastic support, counsel, and patience throughout the past two years.

# ESSAYS

# WOMEN IN SCIENCE THROUGHOUT HISTORY

MARILYN BAILEY OGILVIE, PH.D.

Not many years ago if a person was asked to name some important women scientists he/she might look puzzled at first but eventually might come up with the name of only one woman, Marie Curie. It was widely believed that women and science were incompatible, and did not mesh with accepted ideas of feminine nature. There were rarities such as Marie Curie, but the general assumption was that women scientists were virtually non-existent. However, from the 1970s with the passage of the Equal Employment Opportunity Act in the United States and the advent of the women's movement the idea that women either were uninterested or incapable of doing serious science was challenged. Feminists and historians of science set about to find "lost" female scientists and came up with a surprising number. Only after they were "found" could the process of interpreting their lives and works begin. The search yielded evidence that women had been a part of the scientific enterprise from antiquity to the present. An era of collecting the scant available information resulted in a number of biographical dictionaries, but data on early women scientists was especially hard to come by. Although this research made it clear that women were involved in certain aspects of the scientific enterprise it also confirmed that their numbers were minimal and that little information was available on the nature of their contributions.

Throughout history the lack of women scientists was explained in one of two contrary ways – either women were not suited by nature to be scientists or their training and education made it difficult for them to succeed in scientific fields. On the nature side, Aristotle (384–322 BCE) blamed woman's intellectual disability on her passive nature for "the female, in fact, is female on account of an inability of a sort *viz,* it lacks the power to concoct semen . . . Femaleness would be considered a 'deformity,' though one which occurs in the ordinary course of nature."[1] A more refined view of the different natures of man and woman was articulated, expanded, and clarified in the work of Enlightenment philosopher Jean-Jacques Rousseau (1712–1778), when he wrote that a perfect man and a perfect woman ought no more to resemble each other in mind than in features. By nature men and women complement each other and going against nature is not only undesirable but futile.[2]

Nurture advocates can also be found in antiquity. Aristotle's teacher, Plato

(424/423 BCE–348/347 BCE) was much more sympathetic to educating women than Aristotle, realizing that it would be a waste of talent to exclude fifty percent of the population. Speaking through Socrates in the *Republic*, Plato speculated that women and men should have similar education. He wrote that no difference in the intellectual natures of men and women had been demonstrated. If either male or female is superior in any "art or pursuit," this task should be assigned to the most fit.[3]

From the material that has survived from the ancient writers, it seems apparent that Aristotle's view was predominant. Nevertheless, the examination of early texts published from even earlier manuscripts revealed that women were mentioned by ancient writers and were involved in the earliest days of science. Although many of these women were involved in the health fields, including the Greek physician Agnodike (last third of the fourth century BCE), others, including Theano (last part of the sixth century BCE, and Hypatia of Alexandria (*ca.* 370–415 CE) were involved in mathematics. During the Middle Ages in the Latin West when science was at a low point, women continued to work in the health areas especially in *materia medica* where we find the fascinating Hildegard of Bingen (1098–1179 or 1180) whose expertise in the therapeutic use of plants as well as her explanation of the workings of the universe were typical of the "science" of that period.

Women's involvement in science was distinctly peripheral during the great burst of scientific creativity that occurred in the sixteenth and seventeenth centuries. However, judging from René Descartes's large number of female correspondents, some women during these times found scientific ideas interesting. Nevertheless, the age that produced Nicolaus Copernicus (1472–1543), Johannes Kepler (1571–1630), Galileo Galilei (1564–1642), William Harvey (1578–1657), Robert Boyle (1627–1691), and Isaac Newton (1642--1727) lacked female equivalents. The explanation for the dearth of women scientists can be found in the culture of the times. Although the scant educational opportunities for women varied considerably from one country to another and from one time to another within the general period, only very privileged women had the opportunity for even a rudimentary education. Nevertheless women such as Margaret Cavendish, Duchess of Newcastle (1623–1673) represented the prototype of the scientific lady in England, and published several works drawing on her understanding of contemporary science. Drawing attention to the poor education of women, Cavendish argued that women were subordinated within the home and limited by the view that they by nature were irrational, incompetent, and unintelligent. On one occasion she blamed women's "stupidity" to be the result of an education such as hers – "women breeding up women, one fool breeding up another; and as long as that custom last there is no hope of amendment, and ancient customs being a second nature makes folly hereditary in that sex."[4]

The nineteenth-century iteration of the "nature" view of women's abilities was the "two spheres" concept. Woman's sphere was the domestic; man's the public. Usually viewed as separate but equal, these gendered spheres were not equal. Indeed, in the 1850s the romantic vision inherited from the Middle Ages supposed that woman's sphere was higher than man's, for it included the religious and spiritual aspects of life. Many nineteenth-century commentators were not negative about educating women, for they saw in education the attainment of the spheres concept. The right sort of education would prepare girls to be better wives, mothers, and teachers. However, much rationalization had to occur in order to explain how women could be scientists. Science was seen as tough, rigorous, rational, impersonal, masculine, competitive, and unemotional – characteristics not associated with females. In terms of nineteenth-century stereotypes a woman scientist was a contradiction in terms. Women scientists were caught between two mutually exclusive stereotypes – as scientists they were atypical women; as women, unusual scientists.

Throughout history, women developed strategies to compete in the male domain of science. The strategy of impersonating men was often used by women and had an ancient origin. An early example of this strategy was the report that two women were students in Plato's academy. Axiothea of Phlius (fl. *ca.* 350 BCE) and Lasthenia of Mantinea (*ca.* 300 BCE) were reported to have dressed as men in order to become members of his entourage. Later, the mathematician Sophie Germain (1776–1831), a subject in this exhibition, wanted to take advantage of the newly established École centrale des travaux publiques – now the École polytechnique – whose faculty included eminent mathematicians. Although women were not allowed to attend lectures, she was able to obtain copies of notes taken during the lectures of the mathematician Joseph Louis Lagrange (1736–1813). As did the regular students at the end of a term, she submitted a paper to Lagrange using the male pseudonym Monsieur LeBlanc. Lagrange publicly praised the work, and after he found out its authorship offered himself as Germain's mentor. She later corresponded with Karl Friedrich Gauss (1797–1855) again under the pseudonym LeBlanc.

Another strategy enabled women to enter science by the backdoor. By choosing fields that could be considered "women's work," women were able to infiltrate science. Home economics seemed especially suitable for women because of its proximity to the private sphere and, best of all, it was not particularly interesting to the public-sphered male! Ellen Swallow Richards (1842–1911), the wife of an engineering professor at MIT, is credited with establishing home economics as a discipline. In 1880, she began to stress chemistry's value to the homemaker. However, as "women's work," its "facts" were not valued nearly as highly as were those created by men in the "hard sciences," and the very success of this discipline helped to harden the gender segregation for future generations. Rather than being accepted for other scientific employment once the pioneers had shown women could handle this work, women found themselves more restricted than ever to "women's work." Since women were finding such good opportunities in home economics, many persons – including the first vocational counselors, a new specialty around 1910 – urged ambitious young women interested in science to study home economics. It was the only field where a woman scientist could hope to be a full professor, department chair, or even a dean in the 1920s and 1930s. Another type of women's work in academe was "hygiene," a field that attracted women physiologists.

Certain other sciences were considered suitable for ladies because they could be done at home. Botany and astronomy were two areas that could both utilize the expertise of amateurs and allow them to remain at home to conduct their observations. Astronomy even offered women the possibility of jobs outside the home. Low-paid jobs as computers at the Harvard College Observatory and the Royal Greenwich Observatory provided women with jobs. Women were hired by the Director Edward Pickering of Harvard (1846–1919) because astronomy was moving away from observation and into the new field of photographic astrophysics. The adoption of the technology of cameras and spectroscopes had great implications for women since it required a different labor force. Pickering needed fewer observers – men's work – and many more assistants – women's work – to classify as cheaply as possible the thousands of photographic plates his equipment was generating.

Popularization was another strategy through which women could approach science. For example, Jane Marcet (1769–1858) wrote a series of introductory science books intended for women and young people. In these books a teacher and her students held conversations on various scientific subjects. In one book, *Conversations on Chemistry*, three people, Mrs. B, the teacher, and her two students, Caroline and Emily, discussed recent advances in chemistry. Her books influenced men as well as women and children. The young Michael Faraday lauded this book throughout his life that, as a young apprentice bookbinder with little formal education, he read in 1810. He credited it with introducing him to electrochemistry.

Scientific illustration also was an acceptable way for women to participate in the scientific enterprise. Marie Lavoisier (1758–1836), for example, illustrated her famous husband's books and probably contributed some of the ideas. An even earlier example is that of the German naturalist Maria Sibylla Merian (1647–1717) who with her two daughters traveled to India and Surinam where she sketched and painted specimens and provided information on the flora and fauna of the regions studied.

Although teaching at the lower levels had long been open to women, it was not until the nineteenth century that higher education became a career option. The founding of the women's colleges in the northeastern United States helped defuse the opposition to women penetrating postsecondary education. These colleges, Vassar (1865), Smith (1875), Wellesley (1875), Radcliffe (1879), Bryn Mawr (1885), Barnard (1889), and Mount Holyoke (1893; begun as Mount Holyoke Seminary in 1837) produced numerous contributors to science and provided jobs for talented women scientists. Maria Mitchell (1818–1889), Vassar's first professor of astronomy, both advanced the knowledge in her discipline and trained a new generation of women astronomers. Cytogeneticist Nettie Maria Stevens (1861–1912) received her Ph.D. degree from Bryn Mawr and taught there for many years. Two among many, Mitchell and Stevens illustrate the importance of the women's colleges in the education of women scientists. Although Europe did not have the equivalents of these institutions and the particulars varied from one country to another, in all of Europe the education of women received more attention in the nineteenth century than it had previously.

Throughout time, one of the most useful strategies for a woman who wanted to be a scientist was to collaborate with a colleague or male relative. The best-known example of such an association was that of Marie Sklodowska Curie (1867–1934) and Pierre Curie (1859–1906). Those who preferred to think that women could not think creatively argued that it was Pierre who was responsible for the major ideas and that Marie was merely an efficient helper and implementer. Indeed her most scientifically creative years were those during which she and Pierre shared ideas; nevertheless, the basic hypotheses – those that guided the future course of investigation into the nature of radioactivity – were hers. By winning the Nobel Prize twice, the first in physics and the second in chemistry, Curie was the only woman to be so honored twice.

Although women still have a long way to go in order to gain parity with men in the sciences, the situation has improved vastly over the years. Looking at the Nobel Laureates in three scientific disciplines: physics, chemistry, and physiology and medicine, dating from Marie Curie's 1903 prize in physics through 2009 when three women won the prize, Ada E. Yonath (b. 1939) (chemistry) and Elizabeth H. Blackburn (b. 1948) and Carol W. Greider (b. 1961) (physiology and medicine), we find sixteen women laureates in these sciences. In addition there are at least four women who were exceptionally talented scientists and might have won the prize but for different reasons did not: Chien-Shiung Wu (1912–1997), Rosalind Elsie Franklin (1920–1958), Emmy Noether (1882-1935), and Lise Meitner (1878–1968).

In the third volume of her trilogy on American women scientists, historian of science Margaret Rossiter is guardedly optimistic about the future role of women in science.[5] She discusses the changing role of women in academia, industry, the federal government, and nonprofit institutions. By the 1990s and first decade of the twenty-first century a few women scientists were rising to top positions. However, she noted that academic institutions, especially research institutions, were slow in following the trends. Two notable examples, Nancy Hopkins's revelations about conditions at MIT in 1999 and Harvard president Lawrence Summers remarks in January 2005, indicate that there is still work to be done. Rossiter was hopeful that the institutions involved as well as others with similar views were sufficiently contrite to ignite the beginning of an institutional transformation.

1. Aristotle. *De generatione animalium* 1.20.728a. 18-29, 4.6.775a.13–15.

2. Jean-Jacques Rousseau. *Emile; ou de l'éducation*.

www.ilt.columbia.edu/pedagogies/rousseau/Contents2.html, Book 5, 1242 1256

(accessed May 17, 2013).

3. Plato. *Republic* 5.3, 451.

4. Douglas Grant. *Margaret the First: A Biography of Margaret Cavendish, Duchess of Newcastle, 1623–1673*. London: University of Toronto Press, 1957.

5. Margaret W. Rossiter, *Women Scientists in America. Forging a New World since 1972*. Baltimore: The Johns Hopkins University Press, 2012.

Marilyn Bailey Ogilvie, Ph.D. recently retired as professor in the History of Science Department and as curator of the University of Oklahoma's History of Science Collection, a preeminent, 95,000-volume library. She is an esteemed authority in the history of the science community with contributions devoted to women in science.

# PAVING ROADS FOR THEMSELVES AND OTHERS: WOMEN IN SCIENCE AND MEDICINE

RANDI HUTTER EPSTEIN, M.D., M.P.H., M.S.

A few years ago, during my children's umpteenth check-up at the pediatrician, my daughter, Martha, turned to me and asked, "Mommy, can't daddies be doctors too?"

It sounded like the punch line of a joke, the complete opposite to the riddle I used to hear when I was in grade school. That one – from the 1970s – went something like this: A father and son are in a car accident and they are raced to the hospital at which point the attending physician cries, "I can't operate on that child. That's my son." In those days, it was tricky to figure out that the doctor could have been a mother too.

And yet, as this exhibit shows, women have been working in medicine as healers and researchers for hundreds of years. Back in the tenth century, the enigmatic Trotula served as professor of anatomy and wrote books about childbirth in the vernacular aiming towards a lay audience, rather than using the standard Latin for an elitist readership. For years, scholars debated whether Trotula, this educated person, could really have been a woman. Finally, they agreed. She was indeed a she. In those days in Salerno, women were allowed to enroll in medical school and she earned the title of professor, taking over her husband's position after his death.[1] In the sixteenth century, Louise Boursier, also the wife of a doctor, became midwife to Queen Marie de Medici and author of several popular books on childbirth.

Fast forward to the modern era, starting, say with Colonial times. The role of women as healers remained but they were limited to motherly sorts of things: birth attendant, midwife, children's doctor. The female-friendly fields. Yet, even those opportunities started to dwindle as soon as these medical specialties transformed from trade to profession.

By the late 1800s, for instance, some women were welcomed into science programs and even received Ph.D.s, but more often then not, they got the degree but not the job afterwards. The thinking was that educated women were a good thing not for the job market but to be smart enough to raise their sons.[2]

The first two decades of the twentieth century ushered in a seemingly paradoxical age of feminism and flappers. Women were starving their way into Chanel couture, squeezing into corsets and at the same time fighting for the right to vote. It was also a time when several of the women's medical colleges shuttered. And, along the same lines, leading doctors fought against this first wave of feminism warning that pushy, career-seeking women were destroying their bodies. They pointed to the inchoate field of hormones and warned women that their studies would force energy to their brains, draining crucial baby-making resources. (The thinking being, it was one or the other: brain or uterus.)

So it is against this background with all sorts of immense barriers that the leading female scientists thrived. There seemed to be two survival strategies, as Margaret Rossiter explained in a 1983 article in *The Bulletin of the American Academy of Arts and Sciences*. Some women railed against the contemporary ethos, pummeling male authorities with letters of indignation about the injustice of it all. They pointed to lower pay, lack of opportunities and restricted admission to graduate programs. Others tried to figure out a way to work within the system, creating female niches within the male-dominated profession. In the former category, for instance, was Christine Ladd-Franklin, a physicist-turned-mathematician, who fulfilled the requirements for a Ph.D. from Johns Hopkins in 1882 but because of her gender was denied the degree. She tried to fight the system, forged ahead with her research and founded a fund to help other women earn graduate science degrees. On the other hand, there was Ellen Swallows Richards, a chemist and the first woman admitted to the Massachusetts Institute of Technology, who later taught there without pay – and without complaining – and subsequently launched the field of home economics in the 1890s. "Perhaps the fact that I am not a radical and that I do not scorn womanly duties but claim it as a privilege to clean up and sort of supervise the room and sew things is winning me stronger allies than anything else," she wrote to her parents.[3]

Sure enough, women – even the non-scientists among them – found clever ways to promote each other. In the late 1800s, Johns Hopkins trustees – desperate for money to endow the medical school – reluctantly accepted funds collected by four wealthy Baltimoreans – Elizabeth King, Mary Elizabeth Garrett, M. Carey Thomas, and Mary Gwinn. Reluctantly, it is said, because the fearsome foursome demanded not only that the school admit women but that women learn side-by-side with the men. Dr. William Welch, a founder and pioneering pathologist, cringed, but was forced to cave to their demands.[4]

Savvy women persisted, though their numbers were meager. By the end of the nineteenth century, five percent of American physicians were women. Small but something considering the climate then. Unfortunately, it was a statistic that barely budged for the next half century. When Dr. Robert Ruben, then professor and chair of otorhinolaryngology at Albert Einstein College of Medicine, spoke to Barnard students in 1971, he reported that 6.7 percent of American physicians were women and that he eagerly anticipated a time by the close of the twentieth century when women would make up at least a quarter of the class.[5] Sure enough, the percentage of women graduates in medicine tripled between 1970 and 1980. By the beginning of the twenty-first century, women made up half of the students in medical school and a quarter of all physicians.[6]

Many of them were leading scientists of the day. Dr. Helen Taussig, a pediatric cardiologist, detected the link between thalidomide and physical birth defects (babies born with flipper arms and legs). Her study prompted the ban of the drug in Europe. Thalidomide was never on the market in the U.S., although it was available to some doctors on an investigational protocol, leading to birth defects among forty Americans. The American ban was thanks to another pioneering female scientist, Frances Kelsey, Ph.D. As a reviewer to the U.S. Food and Drug Administration, she advised the agency against approving the drug because she felt safety data were lacking. Hated at first for her seemingly overly cautious ways, Kelsey became a hero after Taussig's findings. In 1962, President John F. Kennedy presented Dr. Kelsey the President's Award for Distinguished Federal Civilian Service.

Georgeanna Seegar – later to become Georgeanna S. Jones – was another trailblazer in the early twentieth century. As a medical student she had the audacity to question the accepted scientific knowledge that the illusive pregnancy hormone originated in the pituitary. Seegar didn't believe it and asked a professor if she could do her own experiment. Lo and behold, she found the hormone in the placenta and published her findings in *Science*. Her mentor advised her to publish under the manly-sounding name "G. Emory Seegar" fearing that the editors would reject research done by a woman.

Seegar as well as other successful women had supportive husbands to thank for their rare male support. Carl Cori, who won the 1947 Nobel Prize with his wife Gerty Cori for their elucidation of glucose metabolism, turned down several job offers until a university offered professorships to both of them.

To be sure, each of these women who broke into the male domain of science and medicine come from a broad array of backgrounds and have chosen different routes to satiate their intellectual cravings as well as to satisfy their yearning to heal, but they all have one thing in common: moxie. These women have defied the trends, broken barriers, and most importantly, while paving roads for themselves, cleared the territory for women who would follow.

1. Robert Ruben, "An Address to Students at Barnard College," *Journal of the American Medical Women's Association*, vol. 27, no. 5 (May 1972), pp. 1–2.

2. Margaret Rossiter, "Women Scientists in America," *The Bulletin of the American Academy of Arts and Sciences*, vol. 3, no. 36 (March 1983), pp. 10–16.

3. http://libraries.mit.edu/archives/exhibits/esr/esr-rumford.html (accessed September 9, 2012).

4. Gerald Imber. *Genius on the Edge: The Bizarre Double Life of Dr. William Steward Halsted*. New York: Kaplan Publishing, 2010, p. 184.

5. Ruben, op. cit. p. 4.

6. Statistics and Benchmarking Report 2008–2009. https://www.aamc.org/newsroom/reporter/march11/180258/viewpoint_march2011.html and http://www.ama-assn.org/resources/doc/wpc/wimtimeline.pdf (accessed September 9, 2012).

Randi Hutter Epstein, M.D., M.P.H., M.S. is an adjunct professor at Columbia Journalism School and the author of *Get Me Out: A History of Childbirth from the Garden of Eden to the Sperm Bank.*

# THE PHYSICAL SCIENCES

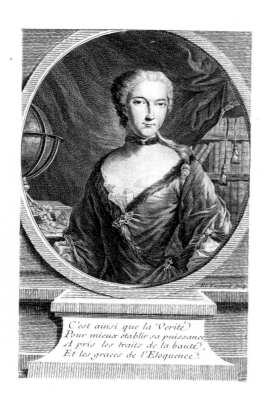

C'est ainsi que la Verité
Pour mieux établir sa puissance
A pris les traits de la bauté,
Et les graces de l'Eloquence.

# INSTITUTIONS
# PHYSIQUES
### DE MADAME LA MARQUISE
# DU CHASTELLET

*adreſſées à Mr. ſon Fils.*

Nouvelle Edition, corrigée & augmentée,
conſiderablement par l'Auteur.

### TOME PREMIER.

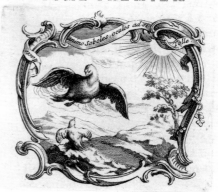

*A AMSTERDAM,*
AUX DEPENS DE LA COMPAGNIE.
M DCC XLII.

Fig. 1. Portrait frontispiece and title page from Émilie Du Châtelet's *Institutions Physiques*, 2nd ed., Amsterdam, 1742. [CAT. 9]

# GABRIELLE-ÉMILIE DU CHÂTELET 1706–1749

## BIOGRAPHY[1]

A unique woman in the scientific community for her background, Gabrielle-Émilie le Tonnelier de Breteuil was born into a family of the minor nobility. Her father was an official at the court of Louis XIV. She grew up in the still-exclusive Place des Vosges in Paris. Self-indulgent, sometimes frivolous, and a source of frequent gossip, she was nevertheless highly intelligent and when she wanted to be, a hard-working scholar. Her early education is undocumented, but by the end of her short life she had demonstrated mastery of advanced mathematics and physics.

An exchange between the connections and wealth of the de Breteuil family and the lineage of a noble family of Lorraine took place with the marriage of Émilie, at age eighteen, to Florent Claude, marquis Du Châtelet, a professional military man. He brought to the marriage only a small château, Cirey. Two children – a daughter who married into a Neapolitan noble family and a son who fell victim to the Reign of Terror[2] – survived Émilie Du Châtelet.

Exactly why, about 1733, Émilie Du Châtelet began the study of advanced mathematics with Pierre-Louis Moreau de Maupertuis and Alexis-Claude Clairaut is unknown. The two men were the leading advocates of Newtonian physics at the Academy of Sciences, and their ideas influenced Émilie Du Châtelet's thinking.[3] Clairaut remained committed to helping her with mathematics for the remainder of her life.

Émilie Du Châtelet and Voltaire became acquainted the same year she began her mathematical studies. Voltaire had returned to Paris in 1729 after two years in London, where he had become enthusiastic about many aspects of life and the tolerant form of government in England. His *Letters Concerning the English Nation* appeared in London in 1733, followed in 1734 by the French edition *Lettres Philosophiques*. Distribution of the French edition led to an arrest warrant, which forced Voltaire into hiding. By the early fall of 1734, Voltaire decided to try life with Émilie Du Châtelet at Cirey, which was sufficiently remote to be ignored by the authorities. Part of the arrangement for his long-term residency at Cirey was funding the restoration of the château. Voltaire lived here, with occasional periods elsewhere, until her death.

Émilie Du Châtelet began reading Newton's *Principia* and English commentaries on the text in 1736. As well, she was helping Voltaire with the text of his book *Elémens de la Philosophie de Neuton*, which appeared in 1738. A careful reading of the *avant propos* in Voltaire's book shows that her contribution to Voltaire's text was substantial and in fact essential. Notwithstanding that she helped write Voltaire's text, she was the author of a lengthy review of his book.[4] By the summer of 1737, she had resolved to proceed on her own to publish in science. The first opportunity she took was the submission – presumably the first by a woman – of an essay for a prize competition of the Academy of Sciences. Voltaire had the same idea and also submitted an essay. Although neither essay was awarded one of the three prizes, both were published in 1739 with the three winning essays.[5] Émilie Du Châtelet published a revised text of her essay in 1744.[6]

By the fall of 1739, Émilie Du Châtelet had begun studying integral calculus, and perhaps indicative of an already-formed plan, she ordered her own copy of Newton's *Principia*. During this time, she was also working on her first book *Institutions de Physique*, published in 1740 and later in an expanded edition in 1742. Her text reveals the problem that most early eighteenth-century French scientists had with Newtonian physics,[7,8,9] to wit, that his physics offered no physical explanation – what was pushing the planets in their orbits around the sun? – for the mathematical equations, which however seemed to give correct answers.

A small publication by Émilie Du Châtelet in 1741 is significant; in it she successfully challenged Dortous de Mairan, secretary of the Academy of Sciences, over the mathematical expression – was it mass times velocity or mass times velocity-squared? – for *forces vives*.[10] Although neither quantity is really a measure of force, her sharp rebuttal, point by point, of de Mairan's arguments, which had appeared in a published letter addressed to her, made him look ineffectual and he retired from the controversy.

Sometime during 1745, Émilie Du Châtelet began her monumental task of translating Newton's *Principia*, with all of its mathematics, into French. The work required four years, and included writing a long commentary and mathematical addendum that she completed shortly before her death in September 1749.[11] The final version of her book, whose exact publication history is mysterious, did not appear until 1759, ten years after her death.

About 1744 Voltaire had begun his well-known affair with his niece, Madame Denis. After some anguish, Émilie Du Châtelet accepted this turn of events, and they continued living together as friends and intellectual companions. In May 1748 her friendship with Jean-François de Saint-Lambert, an undistinguished military officer and poet, turned into a love affair, and she found herself pregnant by February 1749. In April she wrote that she was working seventeen hours a day to finish the mathematical addendum to her translation of Newton.[12] She died on September 10, 1749, ten days after giving birth to a daughter who also did not survive.

## SIGNIFICANT CONTRIBUTIONS

A woman of great intellect, as demonstrated by her achievements in mastering and then writing insightful commentaries on the physics and mathematics of Isaac Newton, Émilie Du Châtelet found herself in the middle of the controversy about Newtonian physics in France. She and Voltaire, outside the academy, were a complement to Maupertuis and Clairaut, the two leading academicians in Paris, in their advocacy of the importance of Newtonian physics.

Her book, to this day, is the only French edition of Newton's *Principia*, and it includes not just her translation with the mathematics, but 287 pages of commentary. In the first section of her commentary, a description of the world and astronomical phenomena is presented without mathematics: she discusses the planetary system, the tides, and the shape of the earth. The latter topic was the most controversial subject within the Academy of Sciences during the early decades of the eighteenth century. Was the earth flattened at the poles as Newtonian physics predicted or was it elongated at the poles, as the French claimed, but later conceded was based upon faulty geodesic data? The second section of her commentary is a formal presentation of the mathematics needed to solve problems about gravitational attraction and the topics discussed in the previous section.

Although Émilie Du Châtelet, as a woman, would not have been considered for membership in the Academy of Sciences in Paris, she had credibility to the extent that, as noted earlier, the Academy's secretary engaged her in a dispute with published texts. That the Academy agreed to publish her prize competition essay was presumably a first for a woman. The Academy of Science of Bologna, having already accepted Laura Bassi as a member,[13] did not hesitate to elect Émilie Du Châtelet to membership in 1746. Émilie Du Châtelet's contributions to physics received little later recognition, an exception being her citation in the article "Newtonianisme" in the *Encyclopédie*.[14]

RKS

## ENDNOTES

1. This section relies mostly on the writings of Judith P. Zinsser, who in 2006 wrote the first satisfying biography of Émilie Du Châtelet. Previous biographies essentially ignore Du Châtelet's scientific work and publications and focus on her love affair with Voltaire.

2. Ken Alder. "Stepson of the Enlightenment: The Duc Du Châtelet, the Colonel who 'Caused' the French Revolution." *Eighteenth-Century Studies*, vol. 32, no. 1 (1998), pp. 1–18.

3. Judith P. Zinsser. "Mentors, the Marquise Du Châtelet and Historical Memory." *Notes and Records of the Royal Society*, vol. 61, no. 2 (May 22, 2007), pp. 89–108.

4. [Émilie Du Châtelet]. "Lettre sur les Elemens de la Philosophie de Newton" (cat. no. 5).

5. *Pieces qui ont remporte Le Prix de l'Academie Royale des Sciences, en M.DCCXXXVIII* (cat. no. 6).

6. [Émilie Du Châtelet]. *Dissertation sur la Nature et la Propagation du Feu*. Paris: Prault, 1744.

7. Carolyn Iltis. "Madame Du Châtelet's Metaphysics and Mechanics." *Studies in History and Philosophy of Science*, vol. 8, no. 1 (1977), pp. 29–48.

8. Linda Garniner Janik. "Searching for the Metaphysics of Science: the Structure and Composition of Madame Du Châtelet's *Institutions de Physique*, 1737–1740." *Studies on Voltaire and the Eighteenth Century*, vol. 201 (1982), pp. 85–113.

9. Sarah Hutton. "Emilie du Châtelet's *Institutions de Physique* as a Document in the History of French Newtonianism." *Studies in History and Philosophy of Science*, vol. 35A, no. 3 (September 2004), pp. 515–531.

10. *Reponse de Madame la Marquise du Chastellet à la Lettre de Mr. de Mairan*. Bruxelles, March 26, 1741. In *Institutions Physiques*, pp. [505]–542 (cat. no. 9). Appended to some copies of the separately issued essay on fire (*supra* 6).

11. Judith P. Zinsser. "Translating Newton's *Principia*: the Marquise Du Châtelet's Revisions and Additions for a French Audience." *Notes and Records of the Royal Society*, vol. 55, no. 2 (May 22, 2001), pp. 227–245.

12. Zinsser, *La Dame d'Esprit*, p. 273.

13. See section on Laura Bassi in this publication.

14. *Encyclopédie*, vol. 22. Geneva: Pellet, 1778, p. 948.

## REFERENCES

Zinsser, Judith P. *La Dame d'Esprit: A Biography of the Marquise Du Châtelet*. New York: Viking, 2006.

Zinsser, Judith P., ed. *Emilie Du Châtelet: Selected Philosophical and Scientific Writings*. Chicago: University of Chicago Press, 2009.

Zinsser, Judith P. and Julie Candler Hayes, eds. *Emilie Du Châtelet: Rewriting Enlightenment Philosophy and Science*. SVEC 2006:01. Oxford: Voltaire Foundation, 2006.

*Madame Du Châtelet: La Femme des Lumières*. Paris: Bibliothèque nationale de France, 2006. Exhibition catalog.

1. Aemilia de Breteuil conjux Marchionis Du Chatellet. [Jean-Marc] Natier pinxit. I. I. Haid fecit et excud. Mezzotint portrait from Johann Jacob Brucker, *Bilder-Sal heutiges Tages lebender und durch Gelahrheit berühmter Schrifftsteller; . . .* , part 4. Augsburg: Johann Jacob Haid, 1745.

From its appearance, the face in this portrait may be based upon that in the frontispiece to the second edition of Du Châtelet's *Institutions Physiques* (1742). Other near-contemporary images of Du Châtelet depict a much more attractive face than seen here. Four pages of text accompany this portrait in Haid's Gallery of Contemporary and Illustrious Learned Authors, which presents Haid's idea of the one hundred most significant European savants of the period.

2. [Voltaire, (François-Marie Arouet, called)]. *Lettres Philosophiques*. Rouen: Jore, 1734. Edition with 26 letters.

Appearing also under the title *Letters concerning the English Nation*, this book, viewed as an attack on French institutions with its praise for many aspects of English society, was the cause of Voltaire's difficulties in 1734. To avoid arrest, he decided to try life with Émilie Du Châtelet in Lorraine, then not a part of France. They lived together at Cirey, the modest Du Châtelet estate, until her death in 1749. The first appearance of the book was an English edition with a London 1733 imprint.

3. [Voltaire, François-Marie Arouet, called]. *Memoirs of the Life of Voltaire*. London: Printed for G. Robinson, 1784.

The first ten pages of these memoirs, translated from a copy of a manuscript that Voltaire had destroyed, provide a touching story of Voltaire's meeting and falling in love with Émilie Du Châtelet: "In the year 1733 I met with a young lady who happened to think nearly as I did, and who took a resolution to go with me and spend several years in the country, . . . This Lady was no other than the Marchioness de Châtelet, who . . . had a mind the most capable of the different branches of science."

4. Voltaire, [François-Marie Arouet, called]. *Elémens de la Philosophie de Neuton*. Amsterdam: Etienne Ledet, 1738.

Although published with only Voltaire's name on the title page, the *avant propos* is clear that Émilie Du Châtelet was in essence a co-author and that her contribution to the text was essential. As Voltaire was in exile from Paris, he gave the manuscript to two publishers in Amsterdam, and two different Amsterdam imprints with the same text are known. Numerous reissues with revisions appeared later. The frontispiece is interpreted as illustrating God's wisdom (the beam of light) coming from Isaac Newton and being reflected by the mirror held by Du Châtelet onto the desk where Voltaire sits putting the ideas into words.

5. [Émilie Du Châtelet]. "Lettre sur les Elemens de la Philosophie de Newton." *Journal des Sçavans*, September 1738, pp. 534–541. Bound volume.

Émilie Du Châtelet's first publication is this eight-page review of the book she helped Voltaire write. Although reviews in this serial are unsigned, she revealed her authorship in a letter to Pierre-Louis Moreau de Maupertuis, a mathematician and friend. Her review emphasizes the significance of Newton's physics and concludes by expressing regret that no one in France has yet produced a comprehensive treatise on physics, such as the many by famous authors in other countries.

6. [Émilie Du Châtelet]. "Dissertation sur la Nature et la Propagation du Feu." In *Pieces qui ont remporte Le Prix de l'Academie Royale des Sciences, en M.DCCXXXVIII*, pp. 85–168. Paris: Imprimerie Royale, 1739.

Du Châtelet's first scientific publication is this essay submitted – presumably the first by a woman – for a prize competition to the Academy of Sciences. Her essay has the sense of a modern scientific paper, with experimental concepts and questions discussed rather than abstract hypotheses posed. She wonders, for example, about the relationships among heat, light, and fire. She observes, mentioning glowworms, that there can be light without heat. Remarkably also, she speculates that different colors may emit different quantities of heat.

The book is printed in *Romain du Roi*, the typeface commissioned by Louis XIV for the exclusive use of the Imprimerie Royale. The typeface can be recognized by the curious lower case L, with its full serif at the top and its small protrusion to the left halfway up the body. Du Châtelet had a revision of the text privately published in 1744, and the Academy reissued the essays in 1752.

7. [Émilie Du Châtelet]. *Institutions de Physique*. Paris: Prault, 1740.

Du Châtelet's text of 1740 was the first new theoretical physics book to appear in France since 1671. She was troubled, as were most French scientists, by the lack of a physical explanation for Newton's mathematical physics, and various metaphysical concepts are introduced. The allegorical frontispiece shows muses of the sciences at the bottom and a female figure climbing to a naked figure, perhaps representing Truth. The figures at the top probably represent Descartes, Newton, and Leibniz.

The inscription "ex dono authoris" on the title page is probably not in Du Châtelet's hand. The signature "Champbonin" on the verso of the title leaf was verified to be that of a close friend of Du Châtelet and Voltaire. M. Champbonin's wife, Anne-Antoinette-Françoise Paulin, Mme de Champbonin, frequently stayed with Voltaire and Du Châtelet as a guest. Mme de Champbonin carried the manuscript of the book to Du Châtelet's publisher in Paris.

8. [Émilie Du Châtelet]. *Institutions de Physique*. Paris: Prault, 1740. With preserved cancellandum.

This copy of Du Châtelet's physics book preserves, tipped-in at the end, a cancellandum, an excised leaf replaced by a new leaf, for pages 313–314. The two pages treat the most controversial topic within the French Academy of Sciences during the early eighteenth century: the shape of the earth as predicted by Newton in opposition to Cartesian opinion in France. Du Châtelet changed her mind about the text on these pages, and had her refined, and more correct, ideas printed for the cancellans, the new leaf inserted during the binding process.

Cancellanda were normally discarded, and preservation of the leaf is a very rare circumstance. The cancellandum was, as usual, slashed to indicate that it was to be removed; the slash was later repaired.

## 9. Madame la Marquise du Chastellet. *Institutions Physiques*. 2nd ed. Amsterdam: aux Depens de la Compagnie, 1742. [SEE FIG. 1]

The second edition of Du Châtelet's physics book has the text enlarged, the addition of documentation about her debate with the secretary of the Academy of Sciences, and a portrait of the author. In contrast to the first edition, her name appears on the title page. The imprint "Amsterdam, aux Depens de la Compagnie" is found in many French books, and its literal reading may not be meaningful. Du Châtelet did not obtain a new permission-to-publish statement for the second edition, perhaps ignoring government regulations, as did Voltaire.

The engraved vignettes at the beginning of each chapter are unusual: although decorative, they depict scenes that relate directly to the topic of each chapter. The chapter about the movement of projectiles has a vignette showing a ball game and a gun and a cannon being fired.

## 10. Madama la Marchesa du Chastellet. *Instituzioni di Fisica*. Venezia: Giambatista Pasquali, 1743.

Du Châtelet's *Institutions de Physique* appeared in 1743 in Italian and German editions, both rare. This Italian example survives in its original stiff paper wrapper, but without the spine. Another "extraordinary woman," Laura Bassi in Bologna, is reported to have used Du Châtelet's book in her classes.

## 11. [Émilie Du Châtelet]. *Du raport des sections coniques par leur generation dans le cosne* (?). With *Du raport des sections coniques par leur description*. Autograph manuscript, ca. 1740. Eight-leaf, stitched gathering from four bifolia; 12 of 16 pages with text, drawings, and equations.

This manuscript seems to be a workbook done in preparation for writing the text on conic sections – circles, ellipses, parabolas, and hyperbolas – in Du Châtelet's translation of Newton's *Principia*. An understanding of the properties of conic sections is essential

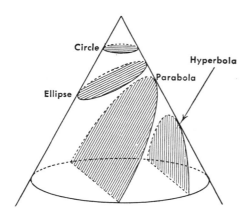

for celestial mechanics, as the orbits of two bodies interacting under Newton's law of gravitation are conic sections. The existence of this manuscript was apparently unnoticed from just after it was written until its discovery in 2010.

12. Émilie Du Châtelet. First bifolium of an eight-page A.L.S. to the Marquis de Saint-Lambert. Paris, June 16, 1748. (Courtesy, The Pierpont Morgan Library, New York.)

In this letter to Jean François de Saint-Lambert, a military officer and poet, with whom Du Châtelet was having a torrid love affair, she alludes to her monumental work in progress, presumably her translation into French of Newton's *Principia*. While sharing her thoughts on love and constancy and forgiving Saint-Lambert for unpleasant words in a previous letter, she communicates a sense of great urgency when discussing her need to finish the book she has been laboring on for two years. Presciently, she writes that her reputation will rest upon this book.

13. Madame la Marquise du Chastellet. *Principles Mathématiques de la Philosophie Naturelle*. 2 vols. Paris: Desaint & Saillant and Lambert, 1759. Ex libris "Bibliothèque du Château de Valençay" with the armorial of Talleyrand and blue stamp "Chateau de Valençay."

During the last few years of her short life, Du Châtelet produced the only French translation – text and mathematics – of Newton's *Principia*. She had copies of both the second (1713) and third (1726) editions of Newton's book for the work. Who arranged for the publication, ten years after her death, of her translation is unknown. Volume two consists mostly of her original writings: a 116-page commentary describing how Newton's work explains celestial mechanics, a 38-page mathematical section, and a 132-page section treating the mathematics of specific problems. The first section of her commentary is based, in part, on Newton's 1731 publication *De Mundi Systemate*. The book exhibited appears in the shelf list of the approximately 16,000 books sold from Talleyrand's library in 1899. The manuscript of her text for volume two was discovered in 2010 and presumably will yield further insights about her work.

# LAURA BASSI 1711–1778

## BIOGRAPHY

In her native city of Bologna, Laura Bassi devoted a lifetime to physics and achieved institutional – as the first woman in Europe to officially hold a university teaching appointment – and international recognition unique for her time. She was the only surviving child of a Bolognese jurist who arranged for her traditional education. In contrast to her contemporary in Milan, Maria Gaetana Agnesi,[1] who had childhood public appearances forced upon her by her father, the first public notice of Bassi occurred when she was twenty, after an academic examination by professors from the University of Bologna and the archbishop of Bologna, the future Pope Benedict XIV.

As a result of her performance during this examination, Bassi became a public figure, and in 1732 ceremonies and disputations were held, along with the award of membership in the Academy of Sciences and the Ph.D. degree by the University of Bologna. Late in 1732 Bassi was given a paid position at the university and she presented her first lecture. Within a short time, she turned to science, and quickly decided to reject Descartes' philosophy in favor of the modern idea that the philosopher's task is "to deduce the laws that govern nature from phenomena observed experimentally."[2]

In 1738 Bassi married fellow scientist Giuseppe Veratti (1707–1793); their prenuptial agreement was to the effect that she could continue her scientific work independently.[3] Frustrated at the restrictions placed on teaching at the university, soon after her marriage Bassi initiated in her home a lecture series, which quickly became a scientific salon. In 1749 Bassi formally organized, also in her home, a school of experimental physics that was attended by students and scholars. Her lectures on experimental physics, which complemented the university's program in theoretical physics, continued for twenty-eight years, almost to the end of her life. Bassi may have used the Italian translation of Emilie Du Châtelet's *Institutions de Physique* in her classes.[4,5,6] Almost 250 pieces of scientific apparatus for experiments in physics are known to have been in the Veratti house.[7]

With the aid of her system of patrons, including Pope Benedict XIV, Bassi achieved further recognition. After some controversy, Bassi obtained the twenty-fifth and last membership in the *Benedettini*, a new category of membership to encourage original research at the Institute of the Academy of Sciences in Bologna. In 1772 the Institute's chair in experimental physics became vacant. As Bassi's husband had been the deceased chair's assistant, he was the logical successor. Among the documents regarding the selection of candidates for the chair of experimental physics is this remark: "finally to satisfy, if one ever can, the demands of Signora Laura Bassi who . . . has asked for this well over three Years, . . . thus it seems that [her request] merits benign attention."[8] In fact, Bassi's husband was passed over and the position of chair went to her. Her husband remained as assistant to her until 1778 when he succeeded to the position upon her death. One of their five surviving children, in turn, briefly held the same position.

SIGNIFICANT CONTRIBUTIONS

Laura Bassi played a leading role in the dissemination of experimental physics in Italy during the middle of the eighteenth century. That she was able for twenty-eight years to maintain an active school of experimental physics suggests the high level of interest she must have created. In addition to university students, she had a role in the life of numerous important Italian scientists, including Lazzaro Spallanzani, her cousin and author on natural history and physiology, and Luigi Galvani, known for his work on animal electricity later correctly explained by Alessandro Volta, a correspondent with Bassi.

Bassi developed a European-wide network of collaborators and correspondents. In electricity, for example, she engaged with the Parisian Jean-Antoine Nollet who visited her in 1749 and with Giambatista Beccaria from Turin, an author of three treatises on electricity and with whom she collaborated on numerous experiments during his visits to Bologna. Many of these relationships continued by correspondence. Bassi was also a staunch defender of Benjamin Franklin's theory of electricity against Nollet's concepts about electricity.

Perhaps among all of the pre-twentieth-century women in the sciences, only Laura Bassi was able to fully engage in activities that were available to her male counterparts. Circumstances, including gender-independent admission to scientific institutions, were probably unique in Italy. In large part she created her own circumstances by actively promoting herself via a patronage network of friends and acquaintances, including Pope Benedict XIV. As well, Bassi and her husband apparently had adopted a model of gender relationships that was very unusual for the period.

Although Bassi frequently lectured, she published very little. Her significant publications were only the two that appeared in 1757 in the annual publication of the Academy of Sciences in Bologna. Her correspondence, unpublished, remains as a rich source of information.

RKS

ENDNOTES

1. See section on Maria Gaetana Agnesi in this publication.

2. Cavazza,"Laura Bassi." p. [11].

3. Marta Cavazza. "Laura Bassi and Giuseppe Veratti: An Electric Couple during the Enlightenment." *Contributions to Science*, vol. 5 (2009), p. 121.

4. Judith Zinsser. *La Dame d'Esprit.* New York: Viking, 2006, p. 210.

5. Madama le Marchesa Du Chastellet. *Instituzioni di Fisica*. Venezia: Presso Giambatista Pasquali, 1743.

6. See section on Émilie Du Châtelet in this publication.

7. Marta Cavazza. "Laura Bassi e ilsuo Gabinetto di Fisica sperimentale: Realtà e Mito." *Nuncius,* vol. 10, no. 2 (1995), pp. 715–753.

8. Translated and quoted by Findlen, p. 466.

REFERENCES

Findlen, Paula. "Science as a Career in Enlightenment Italy: The Strategies of Laura Bassi." *Isis,* vol. 84, no. 3 (September 1993), pp. 441–469.

Cavazza, Marta. "Laura Bassi." Editor's introduction to Laura Bassi, *Miscellanea*. Bologna Science Classics online. Department of Philosophy, University of Bologna. 137.204.24.205/cis13b/bsc03/intro_opera.asp?id_opera=31 (accessed August 28, 2012).

Bassi-Veratti archives online. http://bassiveratti.stanford.edu/ (accessed May 26, 2013).

Ceranksi, Beate. "Bassi Verati (Veratti), Laura Maria Caterina." In *New Dictionary of Scientific Biography*, vol. 1. Detroit: Charles Scribner's Sons/Thomson Gale, 2008, pp. 202–204.

ITEMS EXHIBITED

14. Lavra Maria Catharina Bassi. Litters pinx. I. Iac. Haid excud. Mezzotint portrait from Johann Jacob Brucker, *Bilder-sal heutiges Tages lebender und durch Gelahrheit berühmter Schrifftsteller; . . .*, part 4. Augsburg: Johann Jacob Haid, 1745.

Bassi is depicted with the silver crown of laurels presented upon achievement of the Ph.D. in 1732 from the University of Bologna. Five pages of text accompany this portrait in Haid's Gallery of Contemporary and Illustrious Learned Authors, which presents Haid's conception of the one hundred most significant European savants of the period.

15. Laura Maria Catharina Bassi. *Philosophica Studia*. Bononiae: Ex Typographia Laelii a Vulpe, [1732]. (Courtesy, Special Collections Research Center, University of Chicago Library).

The pamphlet lists the topics of the forty-nine theses that Bassi defended against a panel of academicians on April 17, 1732. The theses consist of six on logic, sixteen on metaphysics, eighteen on physics, and nine on the soul. To take up her paid position at the University of Bologna, Bassi had to defend yet another set of theses on June 27, 1732.

16. Laura Bassi. Commemorative medal in bronze. Bologna, 1732. Ant. Lazari Fec. (Courtesy, Department of Special Collections, Stanford University Libraries.)

This medal, struck in bronze and silver versions, commemorated the award of Laura Bassi's Ph.D. at age 21 from the University of Bologna. A bust of Bassi with a laurel crown appears on the obverse; on the reverse is a depiction of Minerva and a second figure as emblems of learning. Antonio Lazari was the mint-engraver in Bologna.

17. Laurae Bassiae. "De Problemate quodam Hydrometrico," pp. 61–73. With "De Problemate quodam Mechanico," pp. 74–79. In *De Bononiensi Scientiaum et Artium Instituto atque Academia Commentarii*, vol. 4. Bologna, 1757. Volume in original wrapper.

Bassi devoted her life to experimental physics and to its dissemination in Italy. In addition to giving university-sponsored lectures for twenty-eight years, she collaborated on experiments with other prominent Italian scientists. Her two notable papers, one on fluid dynamics and one on mechanics, appear in this volume of the proceedings of the Bologna Academy of Sciences, where she held the chair in experimental physics and was a senior academician.

18. Three contemporary color miniatures depicting events in Laura Bassi's life in 1732. Facsimiles. (Courtesy, Archivio de Stato di Bologna.) [SEE FIG.2]

Leonardo Sconzani. *Laura Bassi difende tesi filosofiche in Palazzo Pubblico*. Bologna, 1732.
Leonardo Sconzani. *Laura Bassi riceve le insegne dottorali in Palazzo Pubblico*. Bologna, 1732.
Leonardo Sconzani. *Laura Bassi tiene la sua prima lezione nell'Archiginnasio*. Bologna, 1732.

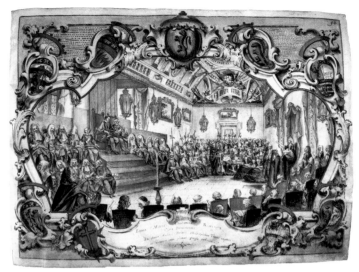

Fig. 2. Contemporary color miniatures depicting events in Laura Bassi's life in 1732. (Courtesy, Archivio de Stato di Bologna.)

TOP: Defense of philosophical theses on April 17.

CENTER: Conferral of her doctoral degree on May 12.

BOTTOM: First lecture at the University of Bologna on December 18.

[CAT. 18]

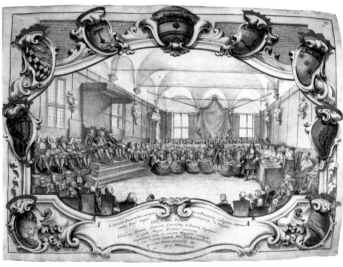

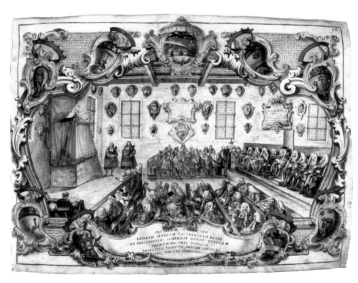

# HERTHA AYRTON   1854–1923

## BIOGRAPHY

Phoebe Sarah Marks – later Hertha Ayrton, an electrical engineer and a prominent suffragette – was the daughter of a Polish Jewish watchmaker and an English mother. Although circumstances were difficult, she received a good education. At the age of sixteen she became self-sufficient, and about this time adopted the name Hertha, earth-goddess, possibly after the poem by A. C. Swinburne. Of great consequence was a chance meeting in 1873 with Barbara Leigh Smith Bodichon, an artist associated with the Pre-Raphaelites, an activist for women's rights, and a co-founder of Girton College, Cambridge. Bodichon supported Hertha Marks from 1877 to 1881 to study mathematics at Cambridge and became a lifelong friend.

After Girton, Hertha Marks taught mathematics privately in London. In 1883 she invented a drawing tool, which was manufactured and sold by a London firm.[1,2] At Finsbury Technical College, she attended evening classes under Professor William E. Ayrton, whose specialty was electricity. She undertook advanced study of electricity on her own. In 1885 she married William Ayrton, who firmly believed that women should have equality of opportunity. He supported her continuing scientific work.

After a few years of modest scientific activities and the birth of a daughter, Hertha Ayrton began research about the properties of electric arcs. The first fruit of this labor was a series of papers in an electrical engineering journal. By 1899 her accomplishments led to an invitation to present a paper, probably the first by a woman, at a meeting of the Institution of Electrical Engineers.

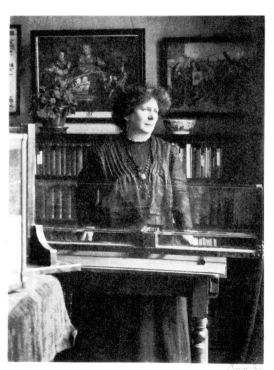

*Mrs. Ayrton in her Laboratory*

Fig. 3. Photograph of Hertha Ayrton, ca. 1908, with experimental apparatus. The portrait is the frontispiece in Evelyn Sharp's biography *Hertha Ayrton 1854–1923: A Memoir* (London, 1926). [CAT. 19]

Later that year she was elected – the first woman – a member of the IEE. In 1900 she was the lone woman to present a paper at the International Electrical Congress in Paris.[3] Her research in electricity culminated in what became the standard text on electric arcs.[4]

Ayrton encountered an unfriendly reception from the Royal Society of London. Her first paper to the Society was read by a member, because a presentation by a woman was not permitted.[5] In 1902 she was proposed for membership in the Royal Society. Her nomination was referred to legal counsel to determine if women were eligible, under the Society's charter, to be considered for membership. A ruling on a more narrow ground was made, to wit, that a married woman was ineligible for membership under the old English common law concept that a married woman had no standing in law. It was 1945 before the first woman was accepted for membership in the Royal Society. In 1904 Ayrton was permitted to read – the first by a woman – a research paper at a Royal Society meeting, and in 1906 she received the Society's Hughes Medal, to date the only woman awardee.[6] Her later publications in the Royal Society's *Proceedings* were devoted to the physics of waves in water with obstacles and boundaries.

Ayrton was deeply involved with the suffragist movement in London. On Black Friday (November 18, 1910) she was "marching immediately behind Mrs. Pankhurst when she entered Downing Street."[7] During the period of arrests and hunger strikes in 1912 and 1913, Ayrton took into her home Mrs. Pankhurst and others released from prison before they died of self-induced starvation. Ayrton was given the funds of the Women's Social and Political Union to prevent them from being seized by the government, and she transferred the money to an account abroad.[8]

Among Hertha Ayrton's friends was Marie Curie.[9] For two months in 1912, Ayrton sheltered Curie and her daughters when Curie was ill and wanted to be out of public view in Paris.[10] Ayrton's social activism for women's rights seems to have had little or no influence on Curie.

A curious *roman à clef* by Ayrton's stepdaughter appeared in 1924.[11] It tells the story of a woman chemist trying to overcome gender bias and gain recognition for her scientific work. On one point, at least, the stories differ: Hertha Ayrton did not have a boyfriend in the British Army during World War I. This part of the fictional story was written to take a swipe at the British government for denying the usefulness, much debated and defended by feminists, of Ayrton's invention of "anti-gas fans" to combat gas attacks in trench warfare.

## SIGNIFICANT CONTRIBUTIONS

Hertha Ayrton's publications represent the work of a modern scientist and a talented electrical engineer. Her research on electricity demonstrated a deep understanding of the non-intuitive characteristics of electricity conducted in arc discharges and led to significant improvements in the operation of arc lighting systems. In particular, she solved the problem of instabilities in arc lighting systems such as were in common use for street lighting. Her 450-page book, filled with graphs and tables of data, was the standard text until the 1920s when newer lighting technologies appeared. The book also provides insights into the curious phenomenon of negative resistance, a very new concept at the time. Her later research about the characteristics of wave motion in liquids and about how the wave motion influences the contours of underwater surfaces have withstood the passage of time.

RKS

## ENDNOTES

1. Sarah Marks. "The Uses of a Line-Divider." *Philosophical Magazine*, s. 5, vol. 19, no. 119 (April 1885), pp. 280–285.

2. William Ford Stanley (cat. no. 20).

3. Hertha Ayrton. "L'Intensité Lumineuse de l'Arc a Courant Continu." In *Congrés International d'Électricité. Rapports et Procès-Verbaux*, International Electrical Congress, Paris, 1900. Paris: Gauthier-Villars, 1901, pp. 250–269.

4. Hertha Ayrton. *The Electric Arc* (cat. no. 21).

5. (Mrs.) Hertha Ayrton. "The Mechanism of the Electric Arc." *Philosophical Transactions of the Royal Society A*, vol. 199 (1902), pp. 299–336.

6. http://royalsociety.org/awards/hughes-medal (accessed April 24, 2012).

7. Sharp, p. 223.

8. Sharp, p. 234.

9. See section on Marie Curie in this publication.

10. Susan Quinn. *Marie Curie – A Life*. New York: Simon & Schuster, 1995, pp. 338–340.

11. Edith Ayrton Zangwill. *The Call*. London: George Allen & Unwin, 1924.

## REFERENCES

Sharp, Evelyn. *Hertha Ayrton 1854–1923*. London: Edward Arnold & Co., 1926.

Mason, Joan. "Hertha Ayrton (1854–1923) and the Admission of Women to the Royal Society of London." *Notes and Records of the Royal Society of London*, vol. 45, no. 2 (1991), pp. 201–220.

Mason, Joan. "Hertha Ayrton (1854–1923)." In *Out of the Shadows*, edited by Nina Byers and Gary Williams. Cambridge: Cambridge University Press, 2006, pp. 15–25.

19. *"Mrs. Ayrton in her Laboratory."* Photograph. London, ca. 1908. Frontispiece from Evelyn Sharp's biography *Hertha Ayrton 1854–1923: A Memoir.* [SEE FIG. 3]

Hertha Ayrton converted the drawing room of her house into a laboratory. Here she is shown with the sand and water tank for her experiments, documented in papers published in 1910, about the formation of sand ripples by waves in water.

20. "Miss Mark's [sic] Space Dividers." In William Ford Stanley, *Mathematical Drawing and Measuring Instruments*, pp. 198–199. [London]: E. & F. N. Spon, 1900.

Hertha Ayrton's first invention, patented when she was still Phoebe Sarah Marks, was an instrument to scale engineering drawings and to do calculations. Her paper about the instrument, which could be used in many more different and unusual ways than similar devices, appeared in 1885 in a scientific journal. Here her device appears in the catalog of a manufacturer of engineering instruments.

21. Hertha Ayrton. *The Electric Arc*. London: "The Electrician" Printing and Publishing Co., [1902].

Ayrton's most important technical publication is this monograph – the contemporary, standard text on the subject. In part, it is a compendium of twelve of her papers published in an electrical engineering journal. Her major contribution was determining the conditions for stable operation of electric arc devices – the first electrical means for lighting. The book is dedicated to Barbara Leigh Smith Bodichon, the artist, feminist, and associate of the Pre-Raphaelites who left a legacy to fund Ayrton's research.

22. *Congrès International. Paris Aout* [sic] *1900*. Photograph.

Hertha Ayrton was the only woman to attend and present a paper at the International Electrical Congress in Paris in 1900. Her twenty-page paper "L'Intensité Lumineuse de l'Arc à Courant Continu" appeared in the conference proceedings. Presumably the lone woman at the far left side of this group photograph of conference attendees is Hertha Ayrton.

23. Hertha Ayrton. Census Form for *Census of England and Wales, 1911*. Facsimile.

Hertha Ayrton was deeply involved with the suffragist movement in London. She marched on Downing Street with Mrs. Pankhurst in 1910 and sheltered suffragettes upon their release from prison after their hunger strikes. Ayrton refused to participate in the 1911 census and wrote across the census form: "How can I answer all these questions if I have not the intelligence to vote between two candidates for parliament? I will not supply these particulars until I have my rights as a citizen. Votes for women. Hertha Ayrton."

24. Hertha Ayrton. "The Origin and Growth of Ripple-mark." *Proceedings of the Royal Society A*, vol. 84, no. 571, pp. 285–310 (October 21, 1910). Offprint.

Ayrton begins this paper – based upon her presentation, the first by a woman, to the Royal Society – by expressing wonder at the ridges and furrows in sand at seashores. She continues by rejecting the current theory about how irregularities in sand form. With a simple experiment, she then demonstrates that oscillatory movement of water over level sand produces a pattern of local accumulation, and she offers an explanation. Further experiments and observations are described.

# MARIE SKLODOWSKA CURIE 1867–1934

## BIOGRAPHY

Poland, under Russian domination, was Marie Sklodowska's home until the age of twenty-four. During this time, Russian policy was to suppress Polish culture and the Polish intellectual class, and her father's career was severely restricted notwithstanding his education. Her mother died when she was ten. A brilliant student, Marie Sklodowska became fluent in Russian and was asked to use this skill when Russian inspectors appeared at her school to verify that only the Russian language was being taught. After completing school, she was employed as a governess for three years. During 1890 she found work in a chemistry laboratory and teaching classes at an underground university in Warsaw.

Late in 1891, Marie Sklodowska moved to Paris and enrolled in science classes at the Sorbonne. By 1894 she had passed examinations in mathematics and physics, and she accepted a research position to investigate the magnetic properties of steel, the subject of her first publication. About this time she met Pierre Curie (1859–1906), already a scientist with important published work, and they married the next year. The first of two daughters was born to the Curies in September 1897.[1]

In seeking a new research subject, Marie Curie apparently had a doctorate in mind – a remarkable idea for a woman at the time. Her attention fixed on the work of Henri Becquerel, who had observed in 1896 photographic plates with exposed areas created by the presence of a uranium-containing mineral. She recognized that Becquerel had made an important scientific observation with a major mystery: what was the source of the energy that exposed the plates?

In late 1897 Marie Curie began an investigation that was the beginning of her life's work. In her first publication in this new field of radioactivity – the Curies's word – she reported that two uranium minerals were much more radioactive than uranium itself could cause, and she concluded, correctly, that there had to be an unknown element in the minerals.[2] Considered in the opposite way, she had discovered that the detection of radioactivity was a method to discover unknown elements.

At this point, his interest raised, Pierre Curie gave up his own research and joined his wife's project. By the middle of 1898 the Curies had isolated a new element, which they named polonium.[4] In December a second new radioactive element, which they named radium, was announced.[5] To confirm the existence of radium by recognized methods, a three-year effort to isolate a quantity of radium and to determine its atomic weight was undertaken. Marie Curie successfully submitted a thesis for a doctorate in 1903. In that year the Nobel Prize in Physics was awarded jointly to Becquerel and to the Curies for their discoveries.

In late 1904 Marie Curie was appointed assistant to Pierre at the Sorbonne. Sadly, their life together ended in early 1906 with the death of Pierre in a street accident. In a biography, the Curies' second daughter wrote in detail about her mother's grief.[5] Marie Curie was named Pierre's successor at the Sorbonne, and for the first time a women held a professorship there. A few years later her first major monograph on radioactivity appeared.[6]

Four events marked Marie Curie's life in 1911. In January she was rejected by the Academy of Sciences for the membership opening; she never attempted again to gain admission. Later in the year she received an invitation to attend, in Brussels, the first of the prestigious Solvay Conferences in Physics. During the conference, Paris right-wing newspapers and scandal sheets chose to expose details, grossly exaggerated, about her affair with Paul Langevin, a married, former Ph.D. student of Pierre's. Two days after the first newspaper accounts of her alleged relationship with Langevin, the Swedish Academy of Sciences awarded Marie Curie a second Nobel Prize, in chemistry this time, for the discovery of polonium and radium. The scandal over her affair with Langevin continued to boil with the publication of letters Curie had written to Langevin, and the Nobel committee suggested that she not attend the award ceremony. Curie promptly rejected that suggestion and appeared in Stockholm to receive the award. The unsavory press reports mostly ended late in 1911.

Marie Curie was active during World War I in organizing a radiological service for the French Army. She oversaw the production of a portable x-ray apparatus for front-line ambulances and the education of doctors in radiology. Her work during the war is described in a small book.[7]

The remainder of Curie's life was devoted mostly to her research laboratory. Her other interests included medical applications of radioactivity, education, fund-raising, and radiation safety. She was late to the recognition of safety matters, and radiation damage was certainly the ultimate cause of her death.

## SIGNIFICANT CONTRIBUTIONS

Marie Curie gave the phenomenon of radioactivity its name and made pioneering use of it in the discovery of previously unknown elements. Her research initiated the field of radiochemistry, and she actively encouraged the industrialization of the science of radioactivity for medical applications. Curie was early to realize that radioactivity was an atomic property of the elements and that it was independent of chemical properties and external factors such as temperature. She was not generally inclined to develop speculative models or mathematical theories for research problems, and she was very cautious about the formulation of general laws to describe her observations. Her English research competitor, Ernest Rutherford, also an experimental scientist and a Nobel awardee, developed many of the concepts relevant to understanding radioactivity and atomic structure.

In all, Marie Curie published about seventy papers. In 1954 the Polish Academy of Sciences published her collected works.[8] She was the first woman to gain an international reputation in science during the twentieth century, and the award of two Nobel Prizes stands as testimony to her accomplishments.

RKS

## ENDNOTES

1. See section on Irène Joliot-Curie in this publication.

2. Sklodowska Curie. "Rayons Émis par les Composés de l'Uranium et du Thorium." *Comptes Rendus*, vol. 126, no. 15 (April 12, 1898), pp. 1101–1103.

3. P. Curie and S. Curie. "Sur une Substance Nouvelle Radio-active, Contenue dans la Pechblende." *Comptes Rendus*, vol. 127, no. 3 (July 18, 1898), pp. 175–178.

4. P. Curie, Mme P. Curie, and G. Bémont. "Sur une Nouvelle Substance Fortement Radio-active, Contenue dans la Pechblende." *Comptes Rendus*, vol. 127, no. 26 (December 26, 1898), pp. 1215–1217.

5. Eve Curie. "*Madame Curie. Garden City, NY: Doubleday, Doran & Co., 1937, chap. 18.

6. Mme P. Curie. *Traité de Radioactivité* (cat. no. 34).

7. Mme Pierre Curie. *La Radiologie et la Guerre* (cat. no. 35).

8. Irène Joliot-Curie, ed. *Oeuvres de Marie Sklodowska Curie*. Warsaw: Académie Polonaise des Sciences, 1954.

REFERENCES

Brian, Denis. *The Curies: A Biography of the Most Controversial Family in Science*. Hoboken, NJ: John Wiley & Sons, 2005.

Quinn, Susan. *Marie Curie: A Life*. New York: Simon & Schuster, 1995.

Reid, Robert. *Marie Curie*. London: Camair Press, 1984.

ITEMS EXHIBITED

25. Marie Curie with apparatus to measure radioactivity. Photograph. Paris, undated. (Courtesy, Rare Book & Manuscript Library, Columbia University.)

26. Marie M. Meloney, Irène Curie, Marie Curie, and Eve Curie. Photograph. United States, 1921. (Courtesy, Rare Book & Manuscript Library, Columbia University.)

Marie M. Meloney was a journalist and the host of Marie Curie's visit to America in 1921 to receive the gift of a gram of radium.

27. *Piezo-electric Quartz Apparatus*. Paris, ca. 1898. (Courtesy, The Mütter Museum of The College of Physicians of Philadelphia.)

The availability of this device – invented by Pierre Curie and his brother Jacques Curie about 1888 and which functions by an electro-mechanical phenomenon called piezo-electricity – was probably a decisive factor in the career of Marie Curie: it was a ready-made device that could be augmented with auxiliary equipment to measure the intensity of ionizing radiation. With this very device Marie Curie characterized the properties of the new radioactive elements she had discovered.

28. Sklodowska Curie. "Recherches sur les Substances Radioactives." *Annales de Chimie et de Physique*, s. 7, vol. 30, pp. 99–144, 145–203, 289–326 (September, October, and November 1903). Bound volume.

About concurrently, Marie Curie's doctoral dissertation appeared both as a University of Paris thesis printing and as this serial publication, which was the form that had widespread circulation. The text covers her work, some already published, up to May 1903. The thesis was reprinted, with minor changes, five times during 1903–1904, and numerous translations appeared.

29. Sklodowska Curie. "Radio-Active Substances." *The Chemical News*, vol. 88, pp. 85–86, 97–99, 134–135, 145–147, 159–160, 169–171, 175–177, 187–188, 199–201, 211–212, 223–224,

Fig. 4. Illustration from the lead article of the November 10, 1906 issue of *L'Illustration,* depicting Marie Curie's first lecture at the Sorbonne. [CAT. 33]

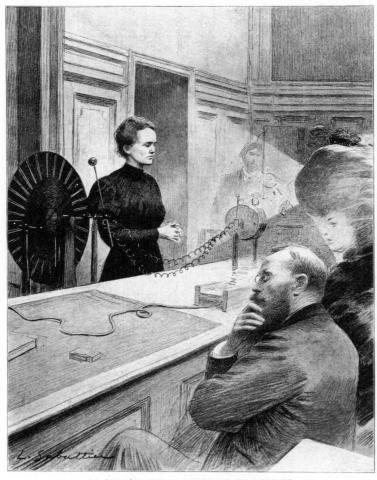

LA PREMIÈRE FEMME PROFESSANT EN SORBONNE

Mme Pierre Curie inaugurant son cours sur la radioactivité. — Au premier rang des auditeurs, M. Appell, Joyen de la Faculté des sciences de Paris.
Dessin d'après nature de L. Sabattier. — Voir l'article à la page suivante (Courrier de Paris).

235–236, 247–249, 259–261, 271–272 (August 21 to December 4, 1903). Bound volume.

This serial edition of Curie's thesis in English is the first translation into any language and is the only translation done from her original thesis text printed in the University of Paris format for her examination committee. After the last installment, the publisher of the journal issued the text as a monograph in late December and reissues appeared in 1904.

30. "Le Laboratoire de la Rue Lhomond." *Le Radium*, year 1, no. 1 (January 1904). Bound volume.

The discoveries of the Curies inspired a new serial, with the Curies pictured on the front page of the first issue. The feature article is a review by Becquerel, whose 1896 papers were the inspiration for Marie Curie's research. *Le Radium* initially appeared in six issues during the first half of 1904. In July 1904 a new serial under the same title by a different publisher appeared; it lasted until late 1919, but with publication suspended during World War I.

31. "Une Nouvelle Découverte – Le Radium: M. et Mme Curie dans leur Laboratoire." *Le Petit Parisien* (January 10, 1904). Single issue.

32. "La Découverte du Radium." *Soleil du Dimanche* (January 17, 1904). Single issue.

Numerous Parisian magazines and newspapers printed depictions of the Curies in 1904 upon the announcement of the Nobel award.

33. "La Première Femme Professant en Sorbonne." *L'Illustration* (November 10, 1906). Single issue. [SEE FIG. 4]

Upon the death of Pierre Curie, Marie Curie was named his successor to the chair of physics. For the first time, a woman held a professorship at the Sorbonne.

34. Madame P. Curie. *Traité de Radioactivité*, 2 vols. Paris: Gauthier-Villars, 1910.

Marie Curie's first major treatise is based upon her lectures at the Sorbonne as professor of physics. Almost 1000 pages in length, the text is the most comprehensive summary of the period. Volume one treats measurements and laboratory practice and volume two describes the nature of radiations and the properties of radioactive substances. Volume one has a portrait in heliogravure of Pierre Curie, whose position at the Sorbonne she occupied after his death in 1906.

35. Mme Pierre Curie. *La Radiologie et la Guerre*. Paris: Félix Alcan, 1921.

Until Marie Curie became involved, the medical service of the French military during World War I ignored diagnostic imaging with x-rays. Curie raised funds to equip vans as mobile radiological units and obtained her own driver's license. Her daughter Irène joined in the work to teach doctors how to use the equipment to image war injuries. This book of 1921 – much rarer than Marie Curie's technical publications – describes her experiences and work during the War.

36. Marie Curie. "Impressions of America." Manuscript, 11 pp., [1921]. (Courtesy, Rare Book & Manuscript Library, Columbia University.)

To receive the gift of radium from funds raised among women in the United States, Marie Curie agreed to visit the United States in 1921 and to participate in ceremonies and receptions. Upon her return to France, she wrote about her impressions of the country.

She was intrigued by the existence of women's colleges and by outdoor sports played by the students, and she remarked upon how American universities created a bond between alumni and the institution. Curie described various formal visits, including to the White House, where the radium gift was formally presented to her.

37. Marie Curie. Academic cap. (Courtesy, Rare Book & Manuscript Library, Columbia University.)

During Marie Curie's 1921 visit to the United States, her host, Marie M. Meloney, thought that Curie should have an academic cap and gown for her appearances at honorary events. However, Curie is reported to have refused to wear the cap, as she regarded it as a nuisance. At least one photograph of Marie Curie bareheaded in an academic procession is known. On occasion, her daughter Irène wore it, as documented in a photograph, when she substituted for her mother at ceremonies.

38. Madame Pierre Curie. *Radioactivité*. 2 vols. Paris: Hermann & Cie, 1935.

Left unfinished at Marie Curie's death, the text of this treatise was completed by Irène Joliot-Curie and Frédéric Joliot. The first section of the book deals with the background topics – ionized gases, electrons, and x-rays – that led to the discovery of radioactivity and the bulk of the text is a comprehensive review of radioactivity, radioactive transformations, and the chemistry and physics of radioactive materials.

39. "Madame Curie." *France – 1947*, September 28, 1947. Single issue.

The magazine contains a review of the American movie starring Greer Garson and Walter Pidgeon. The cover illustration, taken from the film, tends to make Pierre look like the scientist and Marie, an assistant. However, the film is criticized for being titled "Madame Curie" as if the brilliant Pierre Curie was the laboratory assistant.

40. Selection of Solvay Conference group photographs, 1911–1933. Bruxelles: Institut International de Physique Solvay, [1961]. Provenance: set presented to Abraham Pais, 1961.

Besides Marie Curie, who was invited to all of the conferences, Irène Joliot-Curie and the nuclear physicist Lise Meitner were invited to the seventh conference in 1933.

# IRÈNE JOLIOT-CURIE  1897–1956

## BIOGRAPHY

The first child of Pierre and Marie Curie, Irène Curie was born at the very beginning of her mother's research career. Irène's education began in a teaching cooperative, organized by scientific colleagues of the Curies, with an emphasis on science. After the death of her father when she was nine, her grandfather took on a large role in Irène Curie's life for the next four years. Her grandfather may have been the source of her lifelong liberal socialist philosophy.[1]

Irène Curie began university courses in physics in 1914. During World War I, she assisted her mother in the organization and installation of apparatus for x-ray radiography of wounded soldiers. In 1918 at the Institut du Radium she began research work that led, in 1925, to a doctoral thesis about the radiation emitted by polonium, an element discovered by her mother. Also in 1925, Frédéric Joliot joined Marie Curie's laboratory and Irène Curie was assigned to teach him basic experimental techniques with radioactive materials. The next year Irène Curie and Frédéric Joliot married and, just as in the case of her parents, the Joliot-Curies conducted some research jointly. Their daughter, Hélène Langevin-Joliot, believes that growing up with radioactivity as a household topic was important for Irène Curie's decision to devote her working life to the same subject and that "she was not afraid of her mother's fame."[2]

Significant research publications by the Joliot-Curies began to appear about 1932. In that year they reported finding a highly penetrating radiation when polonium and beryllium were in contact, but unfortunately they mis-characterized the radiation; within a matter of weeks, an English scientist realized their error and made the correct analysis, for which he received the Nobel Prize in physics in 1935. In 1932 an American, Carl David Anderson, reported the discovery, in cosmic-ray photographs, of the positron, for which he received the Nobel Prize in 1936, and the Joliot-Curies quickly realized that they probably had produced but had not observed positrons created in their laboratory experiments. In new experiments, the Joliot-Curies were rewarded by a major discovery: the first synthesis of a new radioactive material.[3,4] Their experiment consisted of exposing aluminum to alpha particles, which produced emission of neutrons and positrons, and observing that after removing the source of alpha particles, positrons continued to be emitted;

ultimately they determined that a radioactive isotope of phosphorus had been created. For the discovery that new radioactive materials could be synthesized, the Nobel Prize in chemistry for 1935 was awarded to the Joliot-Curies.

After a short term as secretary of state in the Popular Front government in 1936, Irène Curie resumed research work, now independently of her husband, and she was elected professor at the Sorbonne. During the late 1930s she took up an investigation of uranium bombarded with neutrons and found herself in competition with Otto Hahn and Lise Meitner in Berlin, but the discovery of fission eluded Irène Curie. In late 1945 she was appointed a commissioner of the French Atomic Energy Commission, which Frédéric Joliot headed. After Joliot's dismissal for political reasons during the Cold War, her five-year appointment was not renewed. In 1946 she was named director of the Institut du Radium. Irène Curie was active in peace movements, in women's organizations, and in advocating for the rewards of a life in science.

Just as was the experience of her mother, Irène Curie could not win election to the French Academy of Sciences, which was still not open to women. She did receive many other honors. She died of leukemia, presumably from years of casual handling of radioactive materials.

## SIGNIFICANT CONTRIBUTIONS

Among the scientific achievements of Irène Curie, some with her husband, the discovery that new radioactive materials could be synthesized by laboratory methods was the most significant. This discovery led, first of all, to hundreds of researchers quickly taking up the creation and characterization of radioisotopes, unstable forms of elements that undergo nuclear transformation with the emission of radiation. The discovery spawned practical applications of radiochemistry in just about every field of science and medicine.

Radiochemical methods can deal with unweighably small quantities of materials by detection and measurement of the radiation emitted. Radiopharmaceuticals, for example, are short-lived isotopes that concentrate at specific locations in the body and provide data for imaging, diagnosis, and treatment of cancer. An example is the work of Rosalyn Yalow in the development of radioimmunoassay methods, which depend upon measurement of the radioactive decay rate of a radioactive "tracer" in the body.[5] Numerous medical imaging techniques function by the detection of radiation from short-lived isotopes.

RKS

Fig. 5. Title page of Irène Curie's Ph.D. thesis with signed inscription to friends of the Curie family. [CAT. 41]

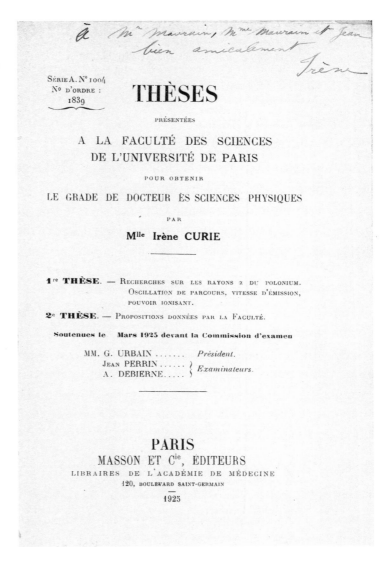

ENDNOTES

1. Perrin, p. 157

2. Langevin-Joliot, p. 142.

3. Irène Curie and F. Joliot. "Un Nouveau Type de Radioactivité." *Comptes Rendus*, vol. 198, no. 3 (January 15, 1934), pp. 254–256.

4. F. Joliot and I. Curie. "Artificial Production of a New Kind of Radio-Element." *Nature,* vol. 133, no. 3354 (February 10, 1934), pp. 201–202.

5. See section on Roslyn Sussman Yalow in this publication.


REFERENCES

Guerra, Francesco, Matteo Leone, and Nadia Robotti. "The Discovery of Artificial Radioactivity." *Physics in Perspective*, vol. 14, no. 1 (March 2012), pp. 33–58.

Langevin-Joliot, Hélène and Pierre Radvanyi. " Irène Joliot-Curie (1897–1956)." In *Out of the Shadows*, edited by Nina Byers and Gary Williams. Cambridge: Cambridge University Press, 2006, pp. 136–148.

Perrin, Francis. "Joliot-Curie, Irène." In *Dictionary of Scientific Biography*, vol. 7. New York: Charles Scribner's Sons, 1973, pp. 157–159.

ITEMS EXHIBITED

41. Irène Curie. *Recherches sur les Rayons a du Polonium*. Paris: Masson et Cie., 1925. Ph.D. thesis, inscribed and signed. [SEE FIG. 5]

Marie Curie's first daughter, Irène, took up her mother's research subject, radioactivity. Beginning studies in 1918, she completed research for a doctorate in 1925. Her thesis reported on the radiation emitted by polonium, one of the elements discovered by her mother. This original printing of Irène Curie's doctoral thesis has an inscription to friends of the Curies – Professor Charles Maurain, his wife, and son – and is signed "Irène."

42. Irène Curie and F. Joliot. *L'Électron Positif*. Paris: Hermann & Cie, 1934.

Irène Curie and her husband, Frédéric Joliot, as collaborators, missed obtaining credit for the discovery of the nuclear particle called the positron. After a report of its discovery by an American scientist, Carl David Anderson, who later received a Nobel Prize, the Joliot-Curies realized that they had produced, but had failed to notice, positrons from their experiments. This missed critical observation prompted their next experiments, reported later in 1934 and which led to a Nobel Prize. In this monograph, the Joliot-Curies provide a brief technical history of positrons.

43. Irène Curie and F. Joliot. "Un Nouveau Type de Radioactivité." *Comptes Rendus*, vol. 198, no. 3, pp. 254–256 (January 15, 1934). Issue in wrapper.

In this paper the Joliot-Curies reported the first laboratory synthesis of a previously unknown radioactive material. After exposing aluminum to one type of radiation for a short time, they observed another type of radiation being emitted later; they found that aluminum atoms had been converted to phosphorus atoms. For the discovery that new radioactive substances could be synthesized, the Joliot-Curies received the Nobel Prize in Chemistry for 1935. This discovery spawned the field of radioisotopes, with its many applications to radiochemistry and radiopharmaceuticals.

44. F. Joliot and I. Curie. "Artificial Production of a New Kind of Radio-Element." *Nature*, vol. 133, no. 3354, pp. 201–202 (February 10, 1934). Issue in wrapper.

To quickly establish priority in the English-speaking world for their discovery that radioactive substances could be created, the Joliot-Curies sent this short note to an English serial with a rapid publication time for important scientific news. They report that the "experiments give the first chemical proof of artificial transmutation" and predict that "other bombarding particles" may also induce nuclear transmutations.

# MARIETTA BLAU   1894–1970

## BIOGRAPHY

Born into an upper middle-class Jewish family in Vienna, Marietta Blau's education enabled her to enroll at the University of Vienna in 1914 to study physics and mathematics. Her Ph.D., awarded in 1919, was based upon research in nuclear physics. In 1921 she joined an x-ray tube factory in Berlin and a year later moved to a staff position at the University of Frankfurt/Main. In 1923 Blau returned to Vienna to care for her ill mother. Excepting two short-term appointments, Blau remained in Vienna at the Institut für Radiumforschung until 1938 – unpaid all this time. It is noteworthy that women constituted about one-third of the researchers at the Institut, probably because of the director's collegial, and apparently gender-independent, management style.

In 1925 Blau began the development of techniques to use photographic emulsions to detect and characterize high-energy particles created by nuclear reactions, and this research topic became her life's work. She worked, in part, with commercial manufacturers to produce emulsions that would permit different nuclear particles to be distinguished and particle energies to be estimated. In 1937, with a student Hertha Wambacher, Blau was the first to observe cosmic ray-induced nuclear reactions with photographic plates.[1]

Blau left Vienna just days ahead of the German annexation of Austria on March 12, 1938. Ellen Gleditsch, a friend of Blau and a former student of Marie Curie, offered Blau a temporary haven in Oslo. Subsequently, Albert Einstein found a position for Blau at a technical university in Mexico, and with her mother she moved there in January 1939. The move to Mexico unfortunately put Blau in exile from research facilities. In Vienna during this period, Blau's former student, Hertha Wambacher, adapted well to the Nazi regime and took Blau's research for her own.

Upon her mother's death, Blau emigrated to the United States in May 1944. Not being adverse to industrial work, she initially found positions with mining companies producing radioactive materials. In 1945 the first description of a scintillation counter with an electronic device to replace the manual counting of scintillations by eye was described,[2] but she did not further develop the technique. In January 1948 a staff position at Columbia University materialized, and while there Blau designed the first apparatus to semi-automatically analyze recorded particle tracks in emulsions,[3] but once again she did not further develop the technique she pioneered.

In 1950 Blau moved to Brookhaven National Laboratory as an employee of the Atomic Energy Commission. In that year Cecil F. Powell was awarded the Nobel Prize in physics in part for the development of photographic methods for particle detection. In the description of his award, one can read much about the prior accomplishments by Blau with no mention of her name.[4] Powell's award emphasized his discovery of the pi-meson, which was an important confirmation of a theoretical prediction. Efforts by two Nobel laureates who nominated Blau for a Nobel Prize went unrewarded, in part at least because she had no effective network of colleagues in the scientific community.

In 1956 Blau received an academic appointment at the University of Miami and government funding for research work. Her health steadily deteriorated, and in 1960 she returned to Vienna to seek care. She quickly discovered that Austrians who had fled in 1938 were not always welcome in Vienna. Surprisingly, however, she returned to research – unpaid – at the Institut für Radiumforschung, but found herself having to deal with former colleagues who had been returned to favor notwithstanding their work under the Nazi regime. The last years of her life in Vienna were perhaps not as satisfying as she had hoped.

## SIGNIFICANT CONTRIBUTIONS

Marietta Blau's pioneering work with photographic methods made the observation of nuclear reactions a simple procedure and permitted the observation of rare nuclear reactions. Her efforts led to the development of optimized photographic emulsions to detect and characterize nuclear particles. Perhaps two opportunities for recognition were missed as she chose not to further develop the method of automating data acquisition from scintillation counters and the apparatus to semi-automatically analyze recorded particle tracks in emulsions. A major limitation to recognition for Blau seems to have been her life-long devotion to one measurement technique and how to improve it. As well, she never became a member of a widespread network of colleagues. The focus of her work seems to have been on method rather than on discovery – not a scientific career path that leads to major recognition and a Nobel award.

RKS

## ENDNOTES

1. M. Blau and H. Wambacher. "Disintegration Processes by Cosmic Rays with the Simultaneous Emission of Several Heavy Particles." *Nature*, vol. 140, no. 3544 (October 2, 1937), p. 585.

2. M. Blau and B. Dreyfus, "The Multiplier Photo-Tube in Radioactive Measurements." *Review of Scientific Instruments*, vol. 16, no. 9 (September 1945), pp. 245–248.

3. Marietta Blau, Robert Rudin, and Seymour Lindenbaum (cat. no. 49).

4. Niels H. de V. Heathcote. *Nobel Prize Winners in Physics 1901–1950.* New York: Henry Schuman, 1953, pp. 452–461.

## REFERENCES

Halpern, Leopold E. "Marietta Blau: Discoverer of the Cosmic Ray 'Stars.'" In Marlene F. Rayner-Canham and Geoffrey W. Rayner-Canham, eds. *A Devotion to their Science.* Montreal: McGill-Queen's University Press, 1997, pp. 196–204.

Strohmaier, Brigitte and Robert Rosner. *Marietta Blau – Stars of Disintegration.* Riverside, CA: Ariadne Press, 2006.

Rentetzi, Maria. "Blau, Marietta." in *New Dictionary of Scientific Biography*, vol. 1. Noretta Koertge, ed., Detroit: Charles Scribner's Sons/Thomson Gale, 2008, pp. 298–302.

Galison, Peter L. "Marietta Blau: between Nazis and Nuclei." *Physics Today*, vol. 50, no. 11 (November 1997), pp. 42–48.

Perlmutter, Arnold. "Marietta Blau's Work After World War II." Unpublished MS., American Institute of Physics, Niels Bohr Library, Manuscript Biographies Collection.

## ITEMS EXHIBITED

45. Marietta Blau with microscope to study particle tracks in photographic emulsions. Photograph. Vienna, before 1938. (Courtesy, Artur Svansson for Agnes Rodhe.) [SEE FIG. 6]

46. Marietta Blau. "Über die photographische Wirkung natürlicher H-Strahlen." *Sitzungsberichte der Akademie der Wissenschaften in Wien*, Mathem.-naturw. Klasse, Section IIa, vol. 134, no. 9 and 10, pp. 427–436, 1 plate (1925). Offprint issued as *Mitteilungen aus dem Institut für Radiumforschung*, No. 179.

Marietta Blau devoted her professional life to the detection and characterization of nuclear particles with photographic emulsions. In this, her first paper on the subject, she reported the detection of protons. Blau is credited with major advances in the technology, later used by many others. Until 1938, when she fled Austria, she had worked unpaid at the Institut für Radiumforschung in Vienna. One of Blau's students adapted to the new regime in Austria and took Blau's work for her own.

47. Marietta Blau. "Bericht über die Entdeckung der durch kosmische Strahlung erzeugten "Sterne" in photographischen Emulsionen." *Sitzungsberichte der Österreichischen Akademie der Wissenschaften*, Mathem.-naturw. Klasse, Section IIa, vol. 159, no. 1 and 2 (1950). Offprint issued as an institutional report, No. Smn 159-7.

Written while she was on the staff of Columbia University, Blau's review paper on cosmic ray stars in emulsions appeared in a post-war publication of the Austrian Academy of Sciences. At the end, discussing her review of the research work, she simply mentions – an amazing understatement for someone forced to flee Austria in 1938 – that the earlier work was interrupted by the political conditions in Austria.

48. M. Blau and J. E. Smith. "Beta-Ray Measurements and Units." *Nucleonics*, vol. 2, no. 6, pp. 67–74 (June 1948). Issue in wrapper.

Upon her arrival in the United States in 1944, Blau found employment with a mining company, where her work focused on measurement methods and instruments for radioactivity. In this paper, the authors point out that the unit of radiation dosage proposed in 1947 as a standard was not suitable for beta rays. Blau and Smith propose the idea of using what later became a standard device, the scintillation counter, and they built one to demonstrate its effectiveness.

49. Marietta Blau, Robert Rudin, and Seymour Lindenbaum. "A Semi-Automatic Device for Analyzing Events in Nuclear Emulsions." *The Review of Scientific Instruments*, vol. 21, no. 12, pp. 978–985 (December 1950). Issue in wrapper.

In this paper Blau and co-workers describe the first concept proposed to automate measurements of radioactivity. She did not continue development of methods to automate data collection, which soon became standard everywhere, and so probably missed an opportunity for enhanced recognition.

50. M. Blau. "Photographic Emulsions." In *Nuclear Physics*, vol. 5, part A of *Methods of Experimental Physics*, pp. 208–264. Luke C. L. Yuan and Chien-Shiung Wu, eds. New York: Academic Press, 1961. With additional articles by Blau: pp. 298–307, 388–408, and 676–682.

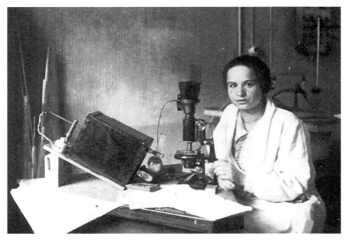

Fig. 6. Marietta Blau, before 1938, Vienna, with a microscope used to reveal tracks of nuclear particles in photographs. (Courtesy, Artur Svansson for Agnes Rodhe.) [CAT. 45]

Thirty-six years after her first publication on the subject, Blau continued to be recognized as the leading authority on the use of photographic emulsions in nuclear and high-energy physics. In this monograph, her four articles provide a comprehensive review of how photographic emulsions can be used to characterize nuclear particles and ionizing radiation.

# LISE MEITNER   1878–1968

## BIOGRAPHY

Lise Meitner – nuclear physicist and co-discoverer of nuclear fission for which an-other scientist, Otto Hahn, received the Nobel Prize – grew up in Vienna in an intellectual and socially liberal family of Jewish origins. Her schooling initially ended, as was the custom in Austria for girls, at age fourteen. However, in 1897 universities were opened to women, and after two years of private study she entered the University of Vienna and earned a doctorate in physics in 1906.

To avoid the only profession, school teacher, open to educated women, Meitner moved to Berlin where she was accepted as a research student by the outstanding theoretical physicist Max Planck. By 1908 Meitner had begun a research collaboration with Otto Hahn, a chemist who specialized in radioactive materials. By 1913 her publication record already listed almost thirty papers, and in that year she became a paid assistant to Planck. For thirteen months during World War I she worked as an x-ray technician, in a role somewhat similar to that of Marie and Irène Curie in France.

Resuming research in late 1916, Meitner did most of the work – although Hahn's name appeared on almost all of the publications and he was given an award for the work – that led to the discovery of protactinium, an element needed to complete a section of the periodic chart of the elements. By 1917 Meitner's reputation was such that she was given the assignment to initiate and head a physics department in the Kaiser Wilhelm Institute (KWI) in Berlin, and by 1920 she had the title of Professor at the KWI. Two years later she qualified – the second woman in Germany – as *Privatdozent*, which meant that she was eligible to be a tenured university professor. By 1926 she was lecturing at the University of Berlin. Among Meitner's accomplishments in Berlin was the observation in 1933 of positrons, the electron's positively-charged equivalent, but her paper appeared fourteen days too late for her to receive credit for the discovery.

In 1934 Meitner initiated, with Otto Hahn and later joined by Fritz Strassmann, the long series of experimental work that led to the discovery of nuclear fission in late 1938. Although the events of 1933 had led to her dismissal from the university, she was able to continue at the KWI because she was an Austrian citizen, and so protected from persecution until 1938. On July 13, 1938 she fled Germany and friends arranged for her to enter, without papers, the Netherlands at a country border station. The day before she fled, the last paper with her name with Hahn and Strassmann had been submitted. Although the collaboration continued by mail, Hahn no longer included her name on publications, probably at first because he felt threatened by the intrusion of Nazi politics into the affairs of the research institute and the possible consequences of his continuing collaboration with Meitner. Later, he seems to have created a narrative that restricted the discovery of nuclear fission to chemistry.

Meitner's circumstances after 1938 were unfortunate.[1] Although given a place in the Nobel Institute for Physics in Stockholm, she was distinctly made unwelcome by the Institute's director. It was here until 1947 that she continued to do experimental work with no help and very modest facilities. Notwithstanding the circumstances, Meitner continued to analyze the experiments being done by Hahn and Strassmann, who did not understand their observations, but reported what seemed to be the presence of a totally unexpected element as a reaction product of the experiments. About Christmas 1939, Meitner, discussing physics with her nephew Otto Frisch, proposed that uranium atoms were being split in the experiments being done by Hahn and Strassmann. A simple experiment by Frisch confirmed the large release of energy she had calculated if a uranium nucleus underwent "fission" – the word introduced into the first paper[2] by Meitner and Frisch – into fragments.

In 1946 Meitner spent six-months in the United States, during which she traveled and taught one semester of nuclear physics at Catholic University in Washington, DC. Upon her return to Sweden, Meitner moved to a technical institute in Stockholm. In 1960 she relocated one last time, to Cambridge, England.

SIGNIFICANT CONTRIBUTIONS

Lise Meitner was a major contributor to modern physics beginning just ten years after the discovery of radioactivity and continuing beyond the discovery of nuclear fission in late 1938. Primarily an experimental physicist, she was especially skilled to exploit the connection between theory and experiment to guide research work. Her research over many years contributed to the completion of radioactive decay series and to the understanding of artificial nuclear reactions, nuclear scattering, and cosmic radiation effects.

Meitner is most well known for her essential part in the discovery of nuclear fission. The story of the 1944 Nobel award in chemistry solely to Otto Hahn for the discovery of fission is a sad tale.[3] Although nominated by former awardees,

Meitner was denied, notwithstanding that she had initiated the project, had been recognized at least by Strassmann as the intellectual leader of the project,[4] and had provided direction for the experimental work done by Hahn and Strassmann. She would not use her life's work for military applications and declined an offer in 1943 to join the Manhattan Project.[5]

RKS

## ENDNOTES

1. Ruth Lewin Sime. "Lise Meitner in Sweden 1938–1960: Exile from Physics." *American Journal of Physics*, vol. 62, no. 8 (August 1994), pp. 695–701.

2. L. Meitner and O. R. Frisch. "Disintegration of Uranium by Neutrons: a New Type of Nuclear Reaction" (cat. no. 53).

3. Elisabeth Crawford, Ruth Lewin Sime, and Mark Walker. "A Nobel Tale of Postwar Injustice." *Physics Today*, vol. 50, no. 9 (September 1997), pp. 26–32.

4. Kraft, p. 834.

5. Sime, p. 305.

## REFERENCES

Kraft, Fritz. "Lise Meitner: Her Life and Times." *Angewandte Chemie International Edition* vol. 17, no. 11 (November 1978), pp. 826–842.

Sime, Ruth Lewin. *Lise Meitner – A Life in Physics*. Berkeley: University of California Press, 1996.

McGrayne, Sharon B. *Nobel Prize Women in Science*. Washington, DC: Joseph Henry Press, 2006.

Watkins, Sallie A. "Lise Meitner: The Foiled Nobelist." In *A Devotion to their Science*, edited by Marlene F. Rayner-Canham and Geoffrey W. Rayner-Canham. Montreal: McGill-Queen's University Press, 1997, pp. 163–191.

## ITEMS EXHIBITED

51. "Lise Meitner (1878–1968), Lecturing at Catholic University." Photograph. Washington, DC, 1946. (Courtesy, Smithsonian Institution Archives. Image 2008-5996.) [SEE FIG. 7]

Meitner made her only visit to the United States during 1946. She was Visiting Professor of Physics at Catholic University, where she taught a course in nuclear physics. During her time in Washington, The Women's National Press Club designated her "Woman of the Year" at a gala event.

52. O. Hahn, L. Meitner, and F. Strassmann. "Ein neues langlebiges Umwandlungsprodukt in den Trans-Uranreihen." *Die Naturwissenschaften*, vol. 26, no. 29, pp. 475–476 (July 22, 1938). Issue in wrapper.

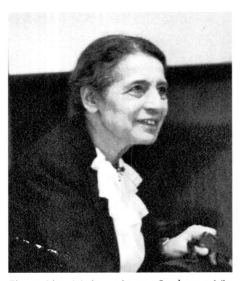

The first paper in the collaboration between Lise Meitner and Otto Hahn, later joined by Fritz Strassmann, appeared in 1935. This 1938 paper was submitted to the journal the day before Meitner, an Austrian of Jewish background, fled Germany. The researchers described their neutron-bombardment experiments in terms of the creation of trans-uranium atoms, and not, as Meitner demonstrated later in 1938, the splitting of uranium atoms.

Hahn's collaboration with Meitner continued by mail, but he did not include her name on later papers, probably at first because he felt threatened by the intrusion of Nazi politics into the affairs of the research institute. Later, he seems to have created a narrative that restricted the research results to chemistry.

Fig. 7. Lise Meitner in 1946 when a Visiting Professor of Physics at Catholic University, Washington, DC. (Courtesy, Smithsonian Institution Archives. Image 2008-5996.) [CAT. 51]

53. L. Meitner and O. R. Frisch. "Disintegration of Uranium by Neutrons: a New Type of Nuclear Reaction." *Nature*, vol. 143, no. 3615, pp. 239–240 (February 11, 1939). Issue in wrapper.

About Christmas 1938, Meitner, living in Sweden, conceived of a nuclear process that could split uranium atoms into fragments of smaller atoms and explain Otto Hahn's experiments. She estimated the energy release expected if a uranium nucleus underwent "fission," and an experiment by her nephew, Otto Frisch, reported in the next issue of *Nature* confirmed the large release of energy. Otto Hahn, alone, received a Nobel Prize for the discovery of fission. The Meitner-Frisch paper is a milestone document for the beginning of the atomic era. Numerous researchers quickly realized that devices based upon fission could release a huge amount of destructive energy.

54. C. Pyle. Lecture Notes. "Taken Feb–June of 1946 at Catholic U. in Washington D.C. by C. Pyle & given by" (signed) Lise Meitner.

Almost 400 students attended Meitner's first lecture in nuclear physics at Catholic University in 1946. More than one hundred completed the course. Clyde Austin Pyle had the clever idea to have Meitner autograph the last page of his lecture notes.

55. Lise Meitner. "The Nature of the Atom." *Fortune*, vol. 33, no. 3, pp. 136–144, 185–186, 188 (March 1946). Issue in wrapper.

*Fortune's* article states Meitner's credentials incorrectly: she did not become a "star in theoretical physics under Dr. Otto Hahn." She was an experimental physicist, also with a Ph.D. but not mentioned, with her own independent department at the Kaiser Wilhelm

Institute, and she, not Hahn, had initiated their joint research program. A chemist and the lone Nobel Prize recipient for the discovery of fission, Hahn did not understand his experimental observations until Meitner provided the explanation.

56. E. Rutherford. *Radioaktive Substanzen und ihre Strahlungen*. Leipzig: Akademische Verlagsgesellschaft m. b. H., 1913. Lise Meitner's copy with signature.

Ernest Rutherford was the leading experimental physicist in radioactivity and nuclear physics in England. Problems under investigation among his many students and collaborators often intersected with Meitner's research. This copy of the German translation of one of Rutherford's books is from Meitner's library with her signature on the title page.

# MARIA GOEPPERT MAYER  1906–1972

## BIOGRAPHY

Maria Gertrud Käte Goeppert was born in the German Empire's province of Silesia, now a part of Poland. She grew up in Göttingen, where her father had an academic appointment, with the understanding that completion of an education to become self-sufficient was expected. For a woman at that time, it is noteworthy that she gained entry to Göttingen University; her original plan had been to study mathematics, but she quickly switched to physics. Her talent was quickly recognized and she became associated with some of Göttingen's most famous research physicists. Her doctoral thesis of 1930 presented a theory of a phenomenon only observed later.

In 1927 the Goeppert household was upset by the death of Maria's father, and her mother took in students as lodgers. One of those students was an American, Joseph Mayer, and in 1930 Maria and Joseph were married and moved to the United States. An academic appointment for her in Germany would have been very difficult to obtain, but, as she discovered, an academic position in the United States was not much easier to obtain, as nepotism rules were common. As well, it may be relevant that no academic institution in the United States had yet shown an interest in her specialty, the application of quantum mechanics to problems in physics and chemistry. Notwithstanding her lack of a formal position, she continued research and published during 1931–1939 while Joseph Mayer held a professorship at Johns Hopkins University. During this time they produced a graduate-level book[1] that was to remain a standard text for decades. While living in Baltimore, the Mayers had two children.

In 1939 Joseph Mayer moved to Columbia University and Maria Mayer found three positions: lecturer at Columbia; part-time teacher at Sarah Lawrence College; and supervisor of a research project at Columbia for the Manhattan Project. Publications from this period list Columbia's Department of Chemistry as her affiliation. In 1946 she joined the newly founded Argonne National Laboratory as Senior Physicist and began an affiliation with the University of Chicago. It was here, with the title "Volunteer Professor"[2] that she did the research that resulted in her 1963 Nobel Prize in Physics for a nuclear shell model that explained the stability of specific atomic nuclei. Mayer was only the second woman, after Marie Curie, to receive the Nobel Prize in Physics. Mayer shared the 1963 Nobel award with J. H. D. Jenson, who independently had developed a model equivalent to Mayer's. In 1955 Mayer and Jensen co-authored a classic text,[3] which Jensen admitted[4] was mostly written by her.

In 1960 both Maria and Joseph Mayer accepted professorships at the University of California, San Diego – her first full-time academic appointment. Unfortunately, shortly after this move, her health was severely affected by a stroke and her research output dropped significantly.

SIGNIFICANT CONTRIBUTIONS

The nuclear shell model was a key discovery for the development of nuclear physics. It explained facts, such as the abundance of specific isotopes of elements that were beyond the predictive capability of the liquid-drop model of nuclei, which treated the particles – protons and neutrons – of atomic nuclei as one ensemble and had been adequate for a basic explanation of fundamental nuclear processes such as fission. Mayer's first step to the shell model was the creation of a detailed summary of data showing that nuclei with "magic numbers" of protons or neutrons were more stable than other nuclei.[5] She then provided an explanation of the origin of the magic numbers by an interaction between the orbital and spinning motions of the protons and neutrons in atomic nuclei, such that a slightly higher binding energy exists between particles in a nucleus with the magic numbers of particles.[6] Thus Mayer's independent particle model yielded an explanation for a large body of experimental information.

That the two models, one collective particle and one independent particle, seem contradictory and only explain specific observations suggested that they represent extreme cases of a more general model, which was developed by others a few years after Mayer's important contribution to nuclear physics.

RKS

## ENDNOTES

1. Joseph Edward Mayer and Maria Goeppert Mayer. *Statistical Mechanics*. New York: J. Wiley, 1940.

2. Moszkowski, p. 209.

3. Maria Goeppert Mayer and J. Hans D. Jensen (cat. no. 60).

4. McGrayne, p. 198.

5. Maria G. Mayer. "On Closed Shells in Nuclei." *Physical Review*, vol. 74, no. 3 (August 1, 1948), pp. 235–239.

6. Maria Goeppert Mayer, "On Closed Shells in Nuclei. II" (cat. no. 59).

## REFERENCES

McGrayne, Sharon B. *Nobel Prize Women in Science*. Washington, DC: Joseph Henry Press, 2006, pp. 175–200.

Moszkowski, Steven A. "Maria Goeppert Mayer (1906–1972)." In *Out of the Shadows*, edited by Nina Byers and Gary Williams. Cambridge: Cambridge University Press, 2006, pp. 202–212.

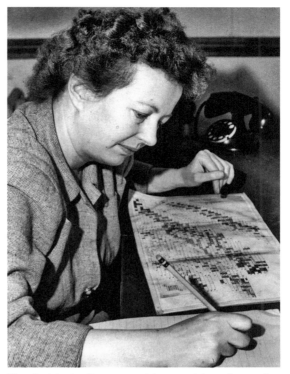

Fig. 8. Maria Goeppert Mayer with a chart of isotopes of the elements. Chicago, undated. (Courtesy, Special Collections Research Center, University of Chicago Library.) [CAT. 57]

## ITEMS EXHIBITED

57. Maria Goeppert Mayer with a chart of isotopes of the elements. Photograph. Chicago, undated. (Courtesy, Special Collections Research Center, University of Chicago Library.) [SEE FIG. 8]

58. Maria Göppert-Mayer. "Über Elementarakte mit zwei Quantensprüngen." *Annalen der Physik*, s. 5, vol. 9, no. 3, pp. 273–294 (1931). Offprint. (Courtesy, Fry's Electronics.)

In her Ph.D. thesis, published as this article, Mayer described the first investigation of atomic phenomena that involve the emission and absorption of two photons (light as a particle carrying energy). Such phenomena had not been observed at the time she did her thesis research. Two-photon processes occur in rare circumstances to conserve energy and angular momentum, and are the basis for certain optical devices.

59. Maria Goeppert Mayer. "On Closed Shells in Nuclei. II." *Physical Review*, vol. 75, no. 12, pp. 1969–1970 (June 15, 1949). Issue in wrapper.

Beginning in the late 1930s, evidence had accumulated to reveal that atomic nuclei with "magic numbers" of protons and neutrons were more stable then others. In this short paper, Mayer provided the explanation with a new model – nuclear shells – for the internal structure of nuclei. She showed that protons and neutrons have a higher binding energy in nuclei with the "magic numbers" of particles. This independent particle model yielded an explanation for many phenomena not explained by the earlier collective particle scheme – the liquid drop model, which could explain fission – of nuclei.

60. Maria Goeppert Mayer and J. Hans D. Jensen. *Elementary Theory of Nuclear Shell Structure*. New York: John Wiley & Sons, 1955.

The authors of this monograph shared the 1963 Nobel Prize in Physics for the nuclear shell model of atomic nuclei. In addition to theoretical work, the book includes a large body of experimental data interpreted with the aid of the shell model. As the second author admitted in a letter, Mayer wrote most of the book.

# CHIEN-SHIUNG WU   1912–1997

## BIOGRAPHY

Born in a small town near Shanghai, C.- S. Wu had the good fortune to have a father so interested in education for girls, then uncommon in China, that he started a school for girls. Wu continued her education at the university in Nanjing, where she majored in physics and had a teacher who had worked with Marie Curie. While a student Wu became a leader of political action groups focused on Chinese nationalism during the turbulent 1930s. After college and working as a research assistant, her supervisor, who had a Ph.D. in physics from the University of Michigan, encouraged her to consider advanced education in physics at Michigan.

With financial help from an uncle, Wu came to San Francisco in 1936. Upon hearing stories of discrimination against women students at Michigan and aware of the reputation of the physics department at the University of California, Berkeley, she enrolled at Berkeley. She completed work for a Ph.D. in 1940, and her first published paper, having to do with nuclear fission, appeared with a future Nobel laureate as co-author.[1] In 1942 Wu married a fellow physicist. Unable at first to obtain an academic appointment at a research university, she took positions as a physics instructor at Princeton University and at Smith College. In March 1944 she moved to Columbia University to work on radiation detectors for the Manhattan Project.

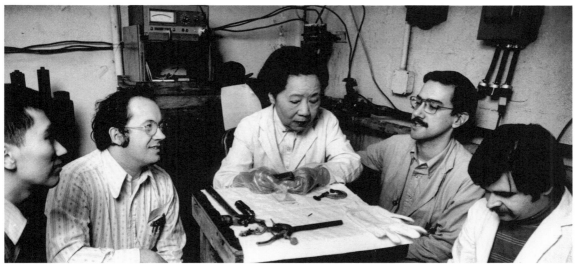

Fig. 9. Chien-Shiung Wu with research students in a Columbia University physics laboratory. New York, undated. (Courtesy, Rare Book & Manuscript Library, Columbia University.) [CAT. 61]

An academic position at Columbia materialized for Wu and she made a sagacious decision to undertake the investigation of beta decay – ejection of an electron from an atomic nucleus that transforms the nucleus into that of a different element – as her primary research topic. At this time in the development of nuclear physics, perhaps no other subject in the hands of a skilled experimentalist could have been more fruitful. Very quickly Wu demonstrated her abilities to select significant problems; to design and build sophisticated apparatus; and to see critical relationships between experiment and theory.

Wu's first major contribution to the physics of beta decay was to produce, in 1949, the first precise measurement of the energy spectrum of emitted beta particles, achieved essentially by the appropriate preparation of the emitting material.[2] In 1956 a major question arose from the deliberations of two theoretical physicists, Chen Ning Yang and Tsung-Dao Lee: was parity – left-and-right-handed, mirror symmetry – conserved in beta decay? Such symmetry is familiar in everyday life and was known to be correct for other nuclear processes. From an experiment carried out with collaborators, to everyone's surprise beta decay did not conserve parity: in essence it was found that different numbers of electrons were emitted in opposite directions with respect to the axis of the atomic nucleus.[3] The experimental proof of the conjecture resulted in an almost immediate Nobel award to Yang and Lee, but not to Wu.

Wu went on to produce many more experimental results that were important for theoretical physics. One of her very unusual investigations applied a 1958 discovery associated with the emission and absorption of gamma radiation by atomic nuclei to important biological questions about blood and sickle cell anemia. During her career at Columbia University she had thirty-three graduate students, an impressive number considering that prospective students knew that she expected them to work long hours seven days a week. Notwithstanding her highly regarded work, she made no independent, major discovery that found favor with a Nobel committee. She received many other major awards, and was the first woman to serve as president of the American Physical Society.

Later in life, Wu's Chinese heritage became important to her. She had maintained contact with the scientific community on Taiwan, and later, after relations between China and the United States were restored, she traveled to the mainland to promote education and to advise on science policy. She voiced her disapproval about repressive Chinese policies and the Tiananmen Square event without jeopardizing her good relations with the Chinese government.

## SIGNIFICANT CONTRIBUTIONS

Without doubt, the research results of Chien-Shiung Wu's work made critical contributions essential for many discoveries in nuclear physics during the second half of the twentieth century. Her selection of beta decay as a research subject was a prescient choice made very early in her career; beta decay was the most mysterious and subtle of the three types – alpha, beta, and gamma – of radioactive decay processes. Her research results on the spectra of beta decay explained former discrepancies, confirmed for the first time Enrico Fermi's theory of beta decay, and was important to complete the understanding of beta decay. The confirmation was important for the acceptance Wolfgang Pauli's concept of the neutrino, which had been proposed, but not experimentally observed, as a mechanism to avoid failure of the law of conservation of energy. Her verification of the non-conservation of parity in beta decay led to the solution of numerous problems in the theory of beta decay. Wu's later work produced yet more important results including a new conservation law and important results for development of a unified theory for electromagnetic and nuclear forces. Her book on beta decay remains the standard work.[4]

RKS

## ENDNOTES

1. E. Segrè and C. S. Wu. "Some Fission Products of Uranium." *Physical Review*, vol. 57, no. 6 (March 15, 1940), p. 552.

2. C. S. Wu and R. D. Albert. "The Beta-Ray Spectra of Cu-64." *Physical Review*, vol. 75, no. 2 (February 1949), pp. 315–316; "The Beta-Ray Spectra of Cu-64 and the Ratio of N+/N-." *Physical Review*, vol. 75, no. 7 (April 1949), pp. 1107–1108.

3. C. S. Wu, et al. "Experimental Test of Parity Conservation in Beta Decay" (cat. no. 63).

4. C. S. Wu and S. A. Moszkowski (cat. no. 64).

## REFERENCES

McGrayne, Sharon B. *Nobel Prize Women in Science*. Washington, DC: Joseph Henry Press, 2006, pp. 254–278.

Wang, Zuoyue. "Wu, Chien-Shiung." In *New Dictionary of Scientific Biography,* vol. 7. Detroit: Charles Scribner's Sons/Thomson Gale, 2008, pp. 363–368.

Wu, Chien-Shiung. "Parity Violation." In *History of Original Ideas and Basic Discoveries in Particle Physics*, edited by H. B. Newman and T. Ypsilantis. New York: Plenum Press, 1996, pp. 381–395.

## ITEMS EXHIBITED

61. C. S. Wu with four research students. Photograph. New York, Columbia University, undated. (Courtesy, Rare Book & Manuscript Library, Columbia University.) [SEE FIG. 9]

62. L. J. Rainwater and C. S. Wu. "Principles of Nuclear Particle Detection." *Nucleonics*, vol. 1, no. 1, pp. 12–23 (September 1947). Issue in wrapper.

Chien-Shiung Wu was initially hired by Columbia University as a research staff member to participate in the development of radiation detectors for the Manhattan Project. Leo James Rainwater, then a Ph.D. student and later the recipient of the 1975 Nobel Prize in Physics, was engaged in similar research. They collaborated and the first issue of *Nucleonics*, a new journal, featured a paper by the two researchers. Rainwater's Ph.D. thesis, and probably their collaborative work, had to be declassified for publication.

63. C. S. Wu, et al. "Experimental Test of Parity Conservation in Beta Decay." *Physical Review*, vol. 105, no. 4, pp. 1413–1415 (February 15, 1957). Issue in wrapper.

This paper reports the first experimental test of a question raised by two theoretical physicists, Chen Ning Yang and Tsung-Dao Lee: is parity – left- and right-handed symmetry, true for other nuclear processes – preserved in the process of electron ejection from an atomic nucleus? The surprising answer determined by Wu and collaborators at a government research laboratory was the negative: the number of electrons emitted in opposite directions with respect to the axis of the nucleus was different. With the question answered, the result was an almost immediate Nobel Prize for Yang and Lee, but not to Wu for answering the question.

64. C. S. Wu and S. A. Moszkowski. *Beta Decay*. New York: Interscience, 1966.

Early in her career, Chien-Shiung Wu made a sagacious decision to undertake the investigation of beta decay – ejection of an electron from an atomic nucleus that transforms the nucleus into that of a different element – as her primary research topic. At the time of her selection of this topic, no other subject in the hands of a skilled experimentalist could have been more fruitful for the future of nuclear physics. It is not surprising, therefore, that she authored what is still the standard monograph on the subject.

65. [C. S. Wu]. Introductory remarks on "Women in Science." Two-page typescript and manuscript, undated. (Courtesy, Rare Book & Manuscript Library, Columbia University.)

Chien-Shiung Wu, growing up in China, had the good fortune to have a father interested in education for girls. Later in life she was very active in encouraging women to take up scientific work, and manuscripts of her presentations on the subject survive. In this short text of remarks at a meeting, she comments on women's progress in science, the roadblocks they face, and strategies to advance the cause of women in science.

# MARIA GAETANA AGNESI 1718–1799

## BIOGRAPHY

The first child, of twenty-one siblings by three mothers, of Pietro Agnesi, a wealthy, ambitious Milanese merchant, Maria Gaetana was recognized very early as a prodigy. Today she is recognized as the first woman to author an advanced textbook of mathematics, including calculus and differential equations. Not yet nine, she delivered in Latin from memory a long oration, by an unknown writer, in defense of women's education.[1] The second child in the family, Maria Teresa, was a skilled musician and composer, whose works are occasionally heard today. The talents of both sisters were often put on display. Although Pietro Agnesi had an enlightened attitude about education for his children, the public activities of the two sisters seem to have been organized to improve the family's social standing.

Until the age of twenty-one, Maria Gaetana participated in academic disputations on natural philosophy in which she defended the "moderns" against the "scholastics." She published, at age twenty-one, a description of almost two hundred theses that she had defended or was prepared to defend.[2]

In 1739 Maria Gaetana Agnesi announced that she wished to retire to a convent.

Her father objected and after negotiations they came to a compromise: she could continue to live at home doing charitable work and mathematics. So her prominent public career ended. She had begun mathematical studies about 1735, and her room in the Agnesi house was filled with mathematical instruments and books by many contemporary scientific authors.[3] Maria Gaetana Agnesi's earliest work on mathematics is a manuscript in the Biblioteca Ambrosiana.

Agnesi's advanced textbook of algebra, geometry, calculus, and elementary differential equations appeared in 1748.[4] It was written neither in Latin nor in her native Milanese language but in the Tuscan dialect, which became the modern Italian language. To produce the book, a printing press was installed in the Agnesi house so that she could supervise the typesetting, a challenge because of the mathematical symbols and complex equations. In some cases, long equations were printed on a large sheet of paper that was folded and inserted into the text. The book was dedicated to Empress Maria Theresa, whose reforms had recently aided the opening of Italian culture to Enlightenment ideas. The title page of the book notes that Agnesi was a member of the Academy of Sciences of Bologna. Shortly after the book appeared, she was offered – but she declined – a formal position in mathematics at the University of Bologna. She also received a congratulatory letter from Laura Bassi, the science lecturer in Bologna.[5]

With her father's death in 1752, Maria Agnesi felt free to pursue her own desires. She began to devote her time to teaching girls from poor families and aiding women in Milan's hospital. From 1771 until her death, she was the director of a large charitable institution. Her sister, Maria Teresa, also felt free upon the death of their father, and she promptly married the man of her choice. In contrast to the other women featured in this publication, Maria Gaetana Agnesi's story is unusual: she gave up scientific work at a young age, thirty-four, and turned to social work for the remainder of her life.

## SIGNIFICANT CONTRIBUTIONS

Agnesi's *Instituzioni Analitiche* is believed to be the first advanced mathematics book by a woman. The text is one of the earliest by anyone to provide a comprehensive introduction to algebra, geometry, differential calculus, integral calculus, and differential equations. The contents, in 1020 pages filled with equations and mathematics, would have been accessible to a wide range of students. Agnesi's book had the particular merit of providing the first formal presentation of Italian terminology for calculus.[6] Her special expertise was the properties of plane curves, which are illustrated on fifty-eight engraved, folding plates.

The significance of *Instituzioni Analitiche* has been discussed by numerous authors with varying opinions. Merit is attached to the fact that Agnesi's book was considered worthy of translation. An English translation was done sometime before 1759 by John Colson at Cambridge and published in 1801. A French translation of volume two was authorized by the French Academy of Sciences and appeared in 1775. It is claimed that *Instituzioni Analitiche* "enjoyed great popularity in Italy."[7] Maria Gaetana Agnesi's book is an early technical book in the Italian vernacular, and has more advanced material than other contemporary European mathematics treatises for young scholars.

RKS

## ENDNOTES

1. Maria Gaetana Agnesi. *Oratio quâ ostenditur; artium liberalium studia à femineo sexu neutiquam abhorrere*. Milan: J. R. Malatestam [1727]. For an English translation, see Messbarger and Findlen, pp. 128–140.

2. Maria Gaetana Agnesi. *Propositiones Philosophicae* (cat. no. 67).

3. Mazzotti. *The World of Agnesi*, p. 102 has a partial list of the scientific authors in her library.

4. Maria Gaetana Agnesi. *Instituzioni Analitiche ad Uso della Gioventù Italiana* (cat. no. 68).

5. See Laura Bassi, *supra*.

6. Findlen, p. 189.

7. Ibid.

## REFERENCES

Findlen, Paula. "Translating the New Science: Women and the Circulation of Knowledge in Enlightenment Italy." *Configurations*, vol. 3, no. 2 (Spring 1995), pp. 167–206.

Mazzotti, Massimo. "Agnesi, Maria Gaetana." In *New Dictionary of Scientific Biography*, vol. 1. Detroit: Charles Scribner's Sons/Thomson Gale, 2008, pp. 19–21.

Mazzotti, Massimo. *The World of Maria Gaetana Agnesi, Mathematician of God*. Baltimore: Johns Hopkins University Press, 2007.

Messbarger, Rebecca and Paula Findlen, eds. and trans. *The Contest for Knowledge: Debates over Women's Learning in Eighteenth-century Italy*. Chicago: University of Chicago Press, 2005.

Truesdell, C. "Maria Gaetana Agnesi." *Archives for History of Exact Sciences*, vol. 40, no. 2 (1989), pp. 113–142.

66. "Maria Gaetana Agnesi." G. B. Bosio, dis. G. A. Sasso, inc. Engraved portrait, early nineteenth century.

During her life Agnesi refused to sit for portraits, so the validity of depictions is unknown. This one is based upon a marble bust, produced by Giuseppe Franchi after visiting her and making a sketch later, in the Biblioteca Ambrosiana.

67. Maria Gaetana Agnesi. *Propositiones Philosophicae*. Mediolani: Joseph Richinum Malatestam, 1738. (Courtesy, The Huntington Library.)

After a formal course of studies, it was common to publish a summary of the subjects studied in the form of theses, which sometimes were defended in public. At age twenty, Agnesi published 191 propositions with short commentaries. She gives mathematics an exalted position among the sciences because it is not subject to fallible empirical knowledge. In the preface, she asserts that women are fit to study the sciences.

68. Maria Gaetana Agnesi. *Instituzioni Analitiche ad Uso della Gioventù Italiana*. 2 vols. Milano: Nella Regia-Ducal Corte, 1748. [SEE FIG. 10]

Maria Agnesi's treatise – 1020 pages filled with mathematics – is one of the earliest comprehensive mathematics books to include calculus and differential equations and is the first mathematics treatise by a woman. Although a native of Milan, she wrote in the Tuscan dialect, the vernacular that became modern Italian. Consequently, her book has the particular merit of defining the terminology for calculus in the Italian language.

To produce the book, a printing press was installed in the family house so that Agnesi could supervise the typesetting – a challenge because of the mathematical symbols and equations. Agnesi's special interest was the characteristics of plane curves, which are depicted on fifty-eight folding plates.

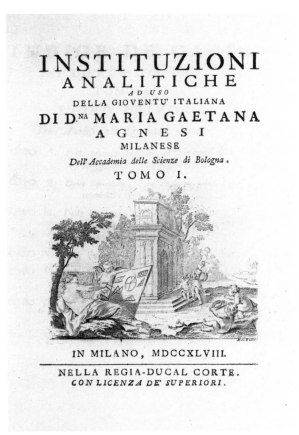

Fig. 10. Title page of Maria Gaetana Agnesi's *Instituzioni Analitiche ad Uso della Gioventù Italiana*, vol. 1 (Milano, 1748). [CAT. 68]

69. Maria Gaetana Agnesi. *Analytical Institutions, in Four Books.* 2 vols. London: Printed by Taylor and Wilks, 1801. Translated by John Colson and edited by John Hellins. (Courtesy, Gerald L. Alexanderson.)

For the use of young scholars, Agnesi's book was more advanced than other contemporary European treatises. The English translator was the Lucasian Professor of Mathematics at Cambridge. Colson's manuscript lay unpublished for almost four decades before a patron, Francis Maseres, was found to fund the costs of editing and printing. The editor was a mathematician and astronomer. By the publication date, the book may have been out-of-date.

70. Maria Gaetana Agnesi. *Traités Elémentaires de Calcul Différentiel et de Calcul Intégral.* Vol. 2. Translated by [Pierre Thomas Antelmy]. Paris: chez Claude Antoine Jombert, 1775.

A copy of Agnesi's *Instituzioni Analitiche* reached the French Academy of Sciences, which issued in 1749 a very favorable report on the second volume, praising it as the best and most complete presentation of calculus and recommending it be translated. The translator, Pierre Thomas Antelmy, a professor of mathematics and an astronomer in a military school in Paris, is not identified in the book.

# MARIE-SOPHIE GERMAIN  1776–1831

## BIOGRAPHY

Marie-Sophie Germain, one of France's renowned mathematicians, was born in Paris, where her father, a silk merchant, was a deputy to the States-General, representing the Third Estate during the time it evolved into the Constituent Assembly. He later became a director of the Bank of France. Germain was only thirteen when her father's library became a refuge from the heady political events of the time. It was there, in J. F. Montucla's *Histoire des Mathématiques,* that the young girl read an account of the murder of the Greek mathematician Archimedes, who was totally engaged in his work during the Siege of Syracuse. Germain decided that she, too, would pursue a career in mathematics. Not surprisingly, she was discouraged by her parents, who considered it unbefitting for a young woman of her time.

A memoir by the mathematician and manuscript thief Guglielmo Libri, who corresponded with Germain, reveals more about her early years. Wrapped in blankets,

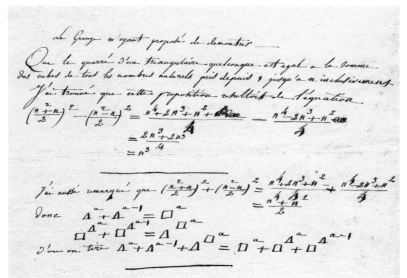

Fig. 11. A manuscript by Sophie Germain demonstrating relationships between sums of triangular numbers and sums of squares. Undated, but ca. 1797. (Courtesy, Gerald L. Alexanderson.) [CAT. 74]

she studied secretly at night despite drastic measures – removal of candles and fire to keep her bedroom dark and cold – taken by her parents to deter their daughter from her obsessive reading habits. Determined and unrelenting, she finally won her parents' approval and support.[1]

She began her studies with geometry and then tackled Latin to read the contributions in physics and mathematics by Leonhard Euler and Isaac Newton. Unable to attend the École polytechnique, which had recently opened but was restricted to males, she succeeded in obtaining copies of lecture notes from a mathematics course taught by Joseph Louis Lagrange. It was customary for students to submit questions and comments at the conclusion of a course. Germain sent her observations to Lagrange under the guise of a male pseudonym, "Le Blanc." Impressed and intrigued by this gifted student, Lagrange was eager to meet his correspondent. Imagine his surprise when he encountered a 20-year-old woman! He soon introduced her to his circle of mathematicians.

Among the mathematicians with whom she corresponded were Adrien-Marie Legendre and Karl Friedrich Gauss. Her letters to Legendre included her work on Fermat's Last Theorem and her observations on Legendre's *Théorie des Nombres* (1798). Legendre incorporated some of her findings in the second edition of his treatise. At the same time, Germain was reading Gauss's *Disquisitiones Arithmethicae*, and later she corresponded with Gauss using her pen name. Gauss did not discover Germain's identity until 1807, when she wrote to him with concern for his well-being during the French occupation of Prussia.[2]

In 1808, when the German physicist Ernst Chladni came to Paris and demonstrated modes of vibrating plates with patterns in sand, Germain turned her attention to these "Chladni figures." In 1811, the French Academy of Sciences offered a prize for a mathematical theory to describe the vibration characteristics of elastic surfaces. Germain submitted a paper using her pen name but did not win a prize until the third and final competition, in 1816. This time she signed her revised paper with her own name. Now 40 years old, she was the first woman to be awarded a prize by the Academy of Sciences. She continued to publish further work on elastic surfaces.[3] Her last publication on the subject was more philosophical than technical and discusses the inadequacies of current theories of elasticity based on molecular forces and is also critical of efforts to reduce physics to mathematics and to find causality embedded in mathematics.[4]

In addition to Sophie Germain's mathematical works, her oeuvre includes several philosophical treatises and poetic meditations, notably *Considérations Générales sur l'État des Science et des Lettres* (1833). This posthumously published work best demonstrates her fundamental belief in the unity of thought between the sciences and the humanities.

In her mature years, Germain developed cancer but continued to work, calling to mind, perhaps, the courageous example set by her childhood hero, Archimedes. She was admired both for her contributions to the sciences and for her tenacity in successfully overcoming gender bias. As Libri recalled in his tribute, Sophie Germain was one of those women who would continue to serve as an example that "the intelligence of their sex is in no way inferior to that of men."[5]

SIGNIFICANT CONTRIBUTIONS

Sophie Germain's scientific work focused on two subject areas: number theory and the mathematical physics of vibrating elastic plates. For the former, which treats the many curious relationships among integers, her lack of a rigorous education in mathematics was not a hindrance, at least initially. Her work in number theory is found recorded in correspondence and in a few published papers and is recognized under the name Germain's Theorem, which deals with the problem of Fermat's Last Theorem. Some of her results appear in a paper by Adrien-Marie Legendre.[6] Much more significant, however, is the recent analysis of previously unstudied manuscripts in which Germain set out a sophisticated research program with new theoretical methods – rediscovered by others later – designed to attack the problem of Fermat's Last Theorem with the goal to produce a comprehensive proof.[7] Much more needs to be done to fully comprehend the contents of these manuscripts. A proof of Fermat's Last Theorem was finally accepted only late in the twentieth century.

In mathematical physics, Sophie Germain's brilliance never reached its potential because she did not have the opportunity to obtain a formal mathematics education. Much of her knowledge came about in a haphazard, unsystematic way, and as viewed from within the community of mathematicians in Paris, she never made the transition from young prodigy to peer. Being a self-taught mathematician with many gaps in her knowledge put her at a significant disadvantage in attempting to apply advanced mathematical analysis to physics problems. Knowing that the necessary mathematical tools for analytical solutions to the vibrating plate problem did not exist, she had the courage – the only person – to enter the prize competition on the subject. Her initial work on the problem yielded important insights on key assumptions relevant to modeling the problem and contributed to the later discovery of the correct mathematical equation. Although her mathematics, as she admitted, was faulty, her results did predict some Chladni figures correctly. Her continuing publications on the problem are best viewed as a part of the scientific process of problem solving that requires fresh ideas and new developments in theory and concept. Today, the need to solve problems about elastic vibrations arises in such diverse fields as structural engineering and electronic device manufacturing. The contributions of Sophie Germain form a part of the very beginning of modern analytical methods for such problems.

PR AND RKS

ENDNOTES

1. Guglielmo Libri. "Notice sur Mlle Sophie Germain." *Journal des Débats*, May 18, 1832. Libri was the Inspector of Libraries in France, during which time he stole thousands of books and manuscripts.

2. Bucciarelli, pp. 24–25, translation of Germain's letter to Gauss.

3. Sophie Germain. *Recherches sur la Théorie des Surfaces Élastiques* (cat. no. 71); Sophie Germain. *Remarques sur la Nature, les Bornes et l'Étendue de la Question des Surfaces Élastiques et Équation Générale de ces Surfaces* (cat. no. 71).

4. Sophie Germain. "Examen des Principes qui peuvent conduire à la Connaissance des Lois de l'Équilibre et du Mouvement des Solides Élastiques." *Annales de Chimie et de Physique*, s. 2, vol. 38 (June 1828), pp. 123–131.

5. Translation by Paulette Rose from: "l'intelligence de leur sexe ne cède en rien à celle du nôtre."

6. [Adrien-Marie] Legendre. "Recherches sur quelques Objets d'Analyse Indéterminée et Particu-

lièrement sur le Théorème de Fermat." *Mémoires de l'Académie Royale des Sciences de l'Institut du France Année 1823*, vol. 6. (Paris: Firmin Didot, 1827), p. 17.

7. Reinhard Laubenbacher and David Pengelley. "'Voici ce que j'ai trouvé:' Sophie Germain's Grand Plan to Prove Fermat's Last Theorem." *Historia Mathematica*, vol. 37 (2010), pp. 641–692.

## REFERENCES

Bucciarelli, Louis L. and Nancy Dworsky. *Sophie Germain: An Essay in the History of the Theory of Elasticity*. Dordrecht: D. Reidel, 1980.

Gray, Mary W. "Sophie Germain (1776–1831)." In *Women of Mathematics: A Bibliographic Sourcebook*, edited by Louise Grinstein and Paul J. Campbell. Westport, CT: Greenwood, 1978, pp. 47–56.

Kramer, Edna E. "Germain, Sophie." In *Dictionary of Scientific Biography*, vol. 5. New York: Charles Scribner's Sons, 1972, pp. 375–376.

Ogilvie, Marilyn Bailey. *Women in Science, Antiquity through the Nineteenth Century. A Biographical Dictionary*. Cambridge: The MIT Press, 1993, pp. 90–92.

## ITEMS EXHIBITED

71. Sophie Germain. *Recherches sur la Théorie des Surfaces Élastiques.* Paris: Mme Ve. Courcier, 1821. [With:]

Sophie Germain. *Remarques sur la Nature, les Bornes et l'Étendue de la Question des Surfaces Élastiques et Équation Générale de ces Surfaces.* Paris: Huzard-Courcier, 1826. (Courtesy, Fry's Electronics.)

These two publications represent Germain's most important work in mathematical physics: the vibration characteristics of elastic surfaces, first noticed in patterns – Chladni figures – formed by sand on a vibrating plate. The research won a prize competition in 1816 sponsored by the French Academy of Sciences. Her contributions to the theory of elastic surfaces came at the very beginning of analytical methods for the study of the vibration characteristics of materials and structures.

72. Sophie Germain. "Examen des Principes qui peuvent conduire à la Connaissance des Lois de l'Équilibre et du Mouvement des Solides Élastiques." *Annales de Chimie et de Physique*, s. 2, vol. 38, pp. 123–131 (June 1828). Issue in wrapper.

In concluding her work about elasticity, Germain published this paper, more philosophical than technical, in which she claims priority for pointing out the inadequacies of current theories of elasticity based on molecular forces. She is also critical of those who tend to reduce physics to mathematics and who seek causality somehow embedded in the mathematics.

73. Sophie Germain. *Oeuvres Philosophiques de Sophie Germain*. Edited by Hte Stupuy. Nouvelle édition. Paris: Firmin-Didot, 1896.

Even without a formal education in mathematics, Sophie Germain contributed to number theory, which treats the many curious relationships among integers. Her work is found mostly in correspondence, printed here. Her early letters to Carl Friedrich Gauss are signed "Le Blanc," and only later did Gauss learn he was corresponding with a woman. She contributed to the problem of Fermat's Last Theorem, finally solved only in 1995.

In addition to Sophie Germain's mathematical correspondence, the volume includes her essay, "Considérations Générales sur l'État des Sciences et des Lettres" (1833), which expresses her fundamental belief in the unity of thought between the sciences and the humanities.

74. Sophie Germain. Mathematical manuscript, one page. Undated, but ca. 1797. (Courtesy, Gerald L. Alexanderson.) [SEE FIG. 11]

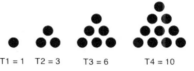

This manuscript illustrates relationships between sums of triangular numbers (1, 3, 6, 10, 15, . . . , which form an equilateral triangle of objects) and squares of numbers. The first equation of the three in the triangle-and-square notation, possibly unique to Germain, reads: the sum of two adjacent triangular numbers is the square of another number. As an example, for the third and fourth triangular numbers, the equation becomes: $10 + 6 = 4^2$. The text goes on to show that a sum of three certain triangular numbers can be expressed as the sum of three squares.

About this manuscript, see Gerald L. Alexanderson. "About the Cover: Sophie Germain and a Problem in Number Theory." *Bulletin of the American Mathematical Society*, n.s., vol. 49, no. 2 (April 2012), pp. 327–331.

# SOPHIE KOWALEVSKI 1850–1891

## BIOGRAPHY

An outspoken nihilist, a woman who flouted social conventions much of her life and wanted a university education, a litterateur, and a mathematician of great accomplishment are perhaps apt descriptors of Sophie Kowalevski.[1] She grew up on a Russian country estate with a sister, Anyuta, and a brother in a family headed by her father, a retired military officer "who had a horror of learned women."[2] In secret, she studied mathematics and physics until her father relented a few years later and permitted formal mathematical studies.

To gain their independence with the goal of a university education abroad, Sophie

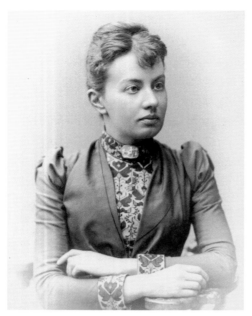

Fig. 12. Sophie Kowalevski. Stockholm, ca. 1889. (Courtesy, Institut Mittag-Leffler.) [CAT. 75]

and Anyuta decided on a radical plan, fictitious marriages. Sophie had the courage to act: she ran away from home to the lodging of Vladimir Kowalevski and sent a note to her father threatening to elope if he did not approve of her marriage to Vladimir. They did marry, in September of 1868, and went first to St. Petersburg and then to Vienna, but neither city had a university that would accept women. By this time, Vladimir was supposed to have disappeared from the sham marriage, but he did not and the result was an unhappy, continuing relationship.

In Heidelberg Kowalevski found that she could attend classes, but that a university degree was not possible. With letters of recommendation, she next applied in Berlin and discovered that classes were not open to women. However, a prominent mathematician, Karl Weierstrass, who although opposed to admitting women to the university, agreed to give her weekly private tutorials. The tutorials continued for almost four years. In 1874 Weierstrass arranged for her to receive a doctorate in mathematics – the first by a woman in Europe – from the University of Göttingen, without ever having presented herself at the university for classes, for examinations, or for a defense of her thesis, which in fact consisted of not one but three significant treatises.

Sophie Kowalevski lived in Russia from 1875 until 1883, and a daughter, Sofya Vladimirovna, was born in 1878. At a mathematics conference in St. Petersburg in 1879 she had the good fortune to meet the Swedish mathematician Gösta Mittag-Leffler, also a former student of Weierstrass; from that meeting Mittag-Leffler was inspired to help Sophie find an academic position. In 1883 the suicide of Vladimir was perhaps a marker for the beginning of a new life. The death of Vladimir ended what had been an unhappy marriage and gave her complete freedom to plan a future.

In 1883 Mittag-Leffler was able to arrange for Kowalevski to begin as a lecturer at Stockholm University. She published important mathematical papers during the next few years and obtained a permanent position at the university. During the last decade of her life, she wrote numerous literary works, many of which had a radical view of political and social affairs in Russia.[3] Only a few of her writings – the most well-known being *The Nihilist Girl* and *Memories of Childhood* – have been translated from the Russian. Unfortunately, in early 1891 at age forty-one, upon her return to Stockholm from a winter holiday in Italy, a bad cold turned into a fatal case of pneumonia. Her daughter was adopted by her godmother in Russia, and Sofya Vladimirovna lived until 1952.

## SIGNIFICANT CONTRIBUTIONS

Considering her somewhat vagabond life and her late start as a mathematician, it is not surprising that Sophie Kowalevski's published output is small, numbering less than a dozen papers. Although her productive professional life was spent outside Russia, she was elected – the first woman – a corresponding member of the Russian Imperial Academy of Sciences.[4] Her work made major contributions in two subjects: the theory of partial differential equations and the theory of motion of rotating bodies in a gravitational field.

Partial differential equations are used to formulate problems involving multiple, independent variables: for example, to write a set of equations describing local temperature as it depends upon time and place, for example, altitude, longitude, and latitude. The Cauchy-Kowalevski theorem, a part of her Ph.D. thesis, became a starting point for future research into the theory of partial differential equations.[5] In particular, her results provided a method to determine the characteristics of solutions to specific types of equations.

The problem of describing the motion of a rotating, arbitrarily shaped body subject to external forces, for example gravity, was recognized three centuries ago as difficult. Only two very specific cases, involving symmetrical objects, had been solved until Sophie Kowalevski's work.[6] She developed solution methods for the more-general case of unsymmetrical rotating bodies, that is, for objects with a center of mass not on the axis of rotation. For this work, begun while she studied with Weierstrass and continued later, she received the Prix Bordin from the French Academy of Sciences, and later, an award from the Swedish Academy of Sciences. Her results became relevant to both theoretical and applied mechanics.

Reviewing the short career of Sophie Kowalevski, one finds that conflicts over gender discrimination did not involve, with one exception, her professional colleagues in mathematics, but rather institutional policies, social expectations, and in some cases professors other than mathematicians. She was accepted as a colleague by most of the other important mathematicians in Europe.

RKS

## ENDNOTES

1. The spelling of her name adopted here is what she used for most of her publications. Other spellings, more directly transliterated from the Russian, are common in the historical literature. In the Items Exhibited list, her name is given as printed in the publications.

2. Kovalevskaya, Sofya. *A Russian Childhood*, p. 6.

3. Koblitz, pp. 257–267.

4. Kovalevskaya, Sofya. *A Russian Childhood*, p. 4.

5. Sophie von Kowalevski. "Zur Theorie der partiellen Differentialgleichungen" (cat. no. 76).

6. Sophie Kowalevski. "Sur le Problème de la Rotation d'un Corps Solide Autour d'Un Point Fixe" (cat. no. 77).

## REFERENCES

Cooke, Roger. "Sonya Kovalevskaya's Place in Nineteenth-Century Mathematics." *Contemporary Mathematics*, vol. 64 (1987), pp. 17–51.

Koblitz, Ann Hibner. *A Convergence of Lives: Sofia Kovalevskaia: Scientist, Writer, Revolutionary*. Cambridge, MA: Birkhäuser, 1983. Reissued: New Brunswick, NJ: Rutgers University Press, 1993.

Kovalevskaya, Sofya. *A Russian Childhood*. Translated and edited by Beatrice Stillman. New York: Springer-Verlag, 1978.

## ITEMS EXHIBITED

**75. Sophie Kowalevski. Photograph, Stockholm, probably 1889. (Courtesy, Institut Mittag-Leffler.)** [SEE FIG. 12]

**76. Sophie von Kowalevski. "Zur Theorie der partiellen Differentialgleichungen."** (*Crelle's*) *Journal für die reine und angewandte Mathematik*, vol. 80, no. 1, pp. 1–32 (1875). Bound volume.

Sophie Kowalevski's first publication – a milestone in the theory of partial differential equations – is based upon her Ph.D. thesis. Partial differential equations are used to formulate problems with multiple independent variables: for example, to write a set of equations for temperature as it depends upon time and location. The Cauchy-Kowalevski theorem provides a method to determine the characteristics of solutions to specific types of equations. The origin of "von" printed with her name is a mystery.

**77. Sophie Kowalevski. "Sur le Problème de la Rotation d'un Corps Solide Autour d'un Point Fixe."** *Acta Mathematica*, vol. 12, no. 2, pp. 177–232 (1889). Issue in wrapper with printed author's inscription added.

This fundamental paper on the subject of non-symmetrical bodies rotating around a fixed point opened up a whole new area of theoretical mathematics. For this work Kowalevski received the prestigious Bordin Prize from the French Academy of Sciences. Before Kowalevski's work, only two special cases of the problem had been solved. With her third solution, it was later shown that no other analytical solutions – not requiring numerical computation – are possible.

78. Sophie Kowalevski. "Sur une Propriété du System d'Équations Différentielles qui Définit la Rotation d'un Corps Solide Autour d'un Point Fixe." *Acta Mathematica*, vol. 14, pp. 81–93 (1890). Offprint. (Courtesy, Fry's Electronics.)

Kowalevski refined the mathematics for which she received the Bordin Prize from the French Academy of Sciences and reported new results in 1890 for which she received an award from the Swedish Academy of Sciences. In part as a result of these awards and also because no one felt able to compete against her, she obtained a lifetime appointment – unfortunately cut short at the age of only forty-one – at Stockholm University. This mathematical work became relevant to both theoretical and applied mechanics as well as to research in mathematics.

# AMALIE EMMY NOETHER  1882–1935

## BIOGRAPHY

The daughter of the mathematician Max Noether, Emmy Noether – one of the eminent mathematicians of the twentieth century – began her education in a way conventional for girls in Germany of her time, and she earned the qualification to teach languages in secondary schools. In 1900 she became interested in mathematics and was allowed to audit classes at the University of Erlangen, where her father was a professor of mathematics. In the fall of 1904 women were permitted to enroll at the university and Noether began work in mathematics for a Ph.D., completed four years later.

Until 1915 Noether continued to live at home, doing research – resulting in ten publications

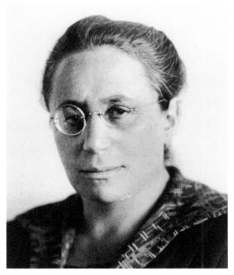

Fig. 13. Emmy Noether, early 1920s in Göttingen. (Courtesy, Special Collections, Bryn Mawr College Library.) [CAT. 79]

and numerous presentations to professional societies – without a position at the university. At the university she sometimes lectured as a substitute for her father and was an advisor for doctoral students.

Emmy Noether was invited by David Hilbert, Germany's leading mathematician, in 1915 to join the mathematics group at the University of Göttingen, the world's center for theoretical mathematics. During the next four years she delivered nine lectures to the Mathematical Society of Göttingen,[1] and in 1918 her milestone paper with the Noether Theorems, important for the development of modern physics, appeared.[2] In 1919 she qualified as a *Privatdozent*, permitting a small salary as an official lecturer; prior to that time her lectures had been announced under Hilbert's name. During the period from 1920 to 1926, she attracted numerous mathematicians and students – she was the doctoral advisor for ten – to her research program and she became a leader in the development of modern abstract algebra. Although academic appointments opened at Göttingen during the period Noether was there, a permanent position was never offered. Nor was she proposed for membership in the Göttingen Academy of Sciences.

After the change of government in April 1933, Noether's permission to teach was rescinded – the usual circumstance for Jewish academics in Germany that year. Fritz Noether, Emmy's brother, also lost his academic position and emigrated to Russia for an academic position in Siberia, where in 1941 he was shot by Soviet authorities for "engaging in anti-Soviet agitation."[3] Later in 1933, Emmy Noether accepted a two-year guest professorship, arranged by The Emergency Committee in Aid of Displaced German Scholars, at Bryn Mawr College. A note in a Bryn Mawr College file mentions her scheduled arrival in New York on the steamship "Bremen" in November 1933.

In early 1934, Noether began a seminar series for a few advanced students at Bryn Mawr, and shortly thereafter some of her former colleagues who resettled at the Institute for Advanced Study at Princeton initiated a weekly lecture series for her at the Institute. Unfortunately, in the spring of 1935 she underwent surgery and succumbed to complications. In a memorial address at Bryn Mawr College by her colleague Hermann Weyl, he mentions in particular "the native productive power of her mathematical genius" and that "her heart knew no malice; she did not believe in evil – indeed it never entered her mind that it could play a role among men."[4]

## SIGNIFICANT CONTRIBUTIONS

Emmy Noether's 1918 paper "Invariante Variationsprobleme" contains the two Noether Theorems, which established a fundamental relationship between symmetries and conservation laws in physics, such that, for example, symmetry properties can be used to search for conservation laws. Such laws in physics – for example, conservation of energy – were traditional assumptions without a fundamental basis, and in the case of one assumed conservation law found, by experiment in 1957, to be incorrect.[5] That energy is conserved in ideal, lossless – for example, without friction – systems is a consequence of the laws of physics being invariant with time. That momentum, the product of mass times velocity, is conserved in ideal systems arises because the laws of physics do not vary with place. Although not appreciated at the time, Noether's theorems were later recognized to be fundamental – although not necessarily used by many physicists – to the development of modern theoretical physics.[6]

Subsequent to her 1918 publication, Noether turned to abstract algebra and indeed she was in large part the founder of this mathematical subject. Her results, the cornerstone for graduate courses in modern algebra, were taken up and converted into the standard text on the subject by one of her students. Algebra, in general, is the mathematics of the rules of operations with objects or sets of objects. "Abstract" in the context of algebra refers to an axiomatic approach to the study of formal properties of operations. Noether's special skill in modern algebra was her ability to extract information of general significance and create universal concepts.

RKS

## ENDNOTES

1. Yvette Kosmann-Schwarzbach. *The Noether Theorems: Invariance and Conservation Laws in the Twentieth Century.* Transl. by Bertram E. Schwarzbach. New York: Springer, 2011, pp. 167–169.

2. Emmy Noether. "Invariante Variationsprobleme" (cat. no. 81).

3. Andrei Parastaev. Letter to H. D. Noether. May 12, 1989. Printed in *Integral Equations and Operator Theory*, vol. 13, no. 2 (March 1990), p. 305.

4. Dick, p. 151.

5. See section on Chien-Shiung Wu in this publication.

6. Nina Byers. "The Life and Times of Emmy Noether: Contributions of Emmy Noether to Particle Physics." In *History of Original Ideas and Basic Discoveries in Particle Physics*, edited by H. B. Newman and T. Ypsilantis. New York: Plenum Press, 1996, pp. 945–964.

REFERENCES

Brewer, James W. and Martha K. Smith, eds. *Emmy Noether: A Tribute to Her Life and Work*. New York: Marcel Dekker, 1981.

Byers, Nina. "Emmy Noether (1882–1935)." In *Out of the Shadows*, edited by Nina Byers and Gary Williams. Cambridge: Cambridge University Press, 2006, pp. 136–148.

Dick, Auguste. *Emmy Noether*. Transl. by H. I. Blocher. Boston: Birkhäuser, 1970.

Kimberling, Clark H. "Emmy Noether." *The American Mathematical Monthly,* vol. 79, no. 2 (February 1972), pp. 136–149.

ITEMS EXHIBITED

79. Emmy Noether. Photograph. Göttingen, early 1920s. (Courtesy, Special Collections, Bryn Mawr College Library.) [SEE FIG. 13]

80. Emmy Noether. "Ueber die Bildung des Formensystems der ternaren biquadratischen Form." Berlin: Georg Reimer, 1908. Separate printing of thesis. Presentation inscription to [Jacob] Luroth. (Courtesy, Fry's Electronics.)

   Noether's thesis work for the Ph.D. was published in the *Journal für die reine und angewandte Mathematik* and as this separatum, similar but not quite identical to the journal publication; which was distributed first is unknown. Her thesis work was a formal computational problem, a type of research once described as very useful for generating Ph.D. theses and to which she never returned.

81. Emmy Noether. "Invariante Variationsprobleme." *Nachrichten von der Königlichen Gesellschaft der Wissenschaften zu Göttingen*. Mathematische-physikalische Klasse. No. 2, pp. 235–257 (1918). Journal issue. (Courtesy, Fry's Electronics.)

   This paper, of great significance for theoretical physics, contains the Noether Theorems, which demonstrate that conservation laws in physics are a consequence of symmetries of time and space. Prior to Noether's work, laws such as the conservation of energy were simply assumed to be true. The paper also resolves a problem in general relativity that Einstein had been unable to solve. Noether was an unpaid assistant and lecturer at the University of Göttingen when this work was done.

82. Emmy Noether to Marion Park. A.L.S. Göttingen, August 18, 1933. (Courtesy, Special Collections, Bryn Mawr College Library.)

   In this letter to the president of Bryn Mawr College, Noether accepts a position in the mathematics department. The position was arranged by the Emergency Committee in Aid of Displaced German Scholars. Edward R. Murrow, before his career as a broadcast journalist, was the organization's assistant secretary who dealt with the paperwork for Noether's appointment. Noether arrived in New York in November 1933.

# FLORENCE NIGHTINGALE 1820–1910

## BIOGRAPHY

Appropriately, "Passionate Statistician" was the sobriquet applied to Florence Nightingale by her first biographer,[1] as she pioneered evidence-based medicine and health care with her statistical work in the second half of the nineteenth century. Her accomplishments came despite growing up in a wealthy English household in which neither a university education nor a profession was expected of women. She did receive, however, a good home-based education, including in mathematics. In 1849 she rejected a proposal of marriage, much to the consternation of her mother, with the feeling that she could not be satisfied "in making society and arranging domestic things."[2]

About the age of sixteen, Florence Nightingale had already decided that she wanted to devote herself to the improvement of the life of the poor and sick, but it was not until 1851 that she was able to take a first step, with the permission of her father, and spend three months at a hospital in Germany. In 1853 her father gave her an annuity and she began work as the superintendent of a small London hospital. A year later the war in the Crimea began, and in October 1854, at the invitation of a family friend, the Secretary at War, which was not a military policy position, she led a team of nurses to the war zone to address the appalling inadequacies of health care in the British Army. Not surprisingly, the Army Medical Department opposed her work. Her accomplishments in the Crimea were enabled only because Nightingale had private sources of funds and had authority independent of the British military.

Upon her return to London in July 1856, Nightingale's career as a statistician and advocate for the use of statistical information for health care began with the data she had collected in the Crimea. Her immediate goals were to reform the Army Medical Department and to identify the causes of mortality in the War. For the latter, it did not take her long to discover that disease due to inadequate sanitary conditions had felled many more soldiers than enemy bullets during the Crimean War, a conclusion that her opposition in the Army Medical Department could not effectively challenge. She engaged William Farr, a physician and statistician, to help, and together during the coming years they produced charts, tables, and graphs to demonstrate the usefulness of statistics as a tool to improve medical care. Nightingale developed a large network of colleagues and advisors in and out of the government. The source of many of her ideas was the Belgian social statistician Adolphe Quetelet, with whom she corresponded.[3]

Nightingale's influence extended as far as to Queen Victoria, and it was the Queen's intervention that created a Royal Commission to respond to Nightingale's data from the Crimean War. Queen Victoria met twice with Florence Nightingale in 1856, and later wrote "I wish we had her at the War Office."[4] As a result of these meetings, the Royal Commission was appointed, and its 600-page report, which included a lengthy text and ten charts by Nightingale, appeared in 1858.[5] Among the illustrations are a number of polar area diagrams, for which she is credited as the inventor.

Nightingale's pioneering work in medical statistics and her effectiveness in putting statistical analysis to use was based upon meticulous data collection, skillful drafting of proposals for action, persuasive presentations, and talent for organization. She regarded statistics based upon research as an organized way to learn from experience. Her goal was to convince officials that statistical analysis provides a rational basis for decision-making processes. Nightingale attempted to get hospitals to adopt a standard form, which she had designed, to collect statistical data. Her proposal of this form was approved at the 1860 International Statistical Congress.[6] However, after just a few years of use in London hospitals, it was abandoned as being "too costly and time consuming."[7]

Mortality of the British Army in India in 1857 was Nightingale's next opportunity to address the failings of the British Army Medical Department, and again she demonstrated that inadequate sanitation was the main cause. From this time until as late as the 1890s, Nightingale devoted much of her efforts to conditions in India, including the analysis of health care data. In 1864 she protested against the Contagious Diseases Acts, pointing out that the role of men in prostitution was ignored. She continued to publish reports based upon her statistical work until well into her seventies, and essentially all of her writings, private and public, are now available.[8]

Florence Nightingale did all of her work as an invalid after 1857, very possibly the chronic aftermath of "Crimean fever," now suspected to have been brucellosis, which nearly killed her in the Crimea. She wrote little during the last ten years of her life. In 1907 she became the first woman to receive Great Britain's highest civilian honor, the Order of Merit.

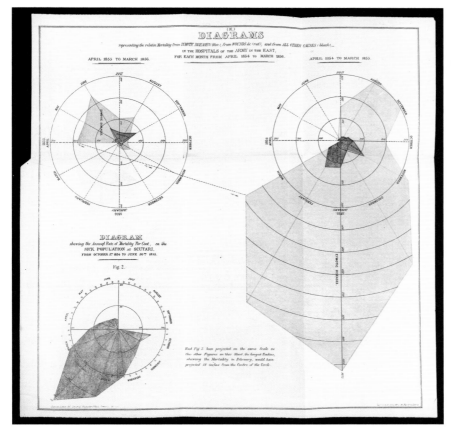

Fig. 14. A polar area diagram, invented by Florence Nightingale and called "coxcombs," to highlight the huge mortality in British military hospitals due to disease, not battle, during the Crimean War, from Report of the Commissioners. . . . London, 1858. The color coding is green for infectious diseases, red for wounds, and black for other causes of mortality. [CAT. 83]

## SIGNIFICANT CONTRIBUTIONS

Usually thought about as the founder of modern nursing as an independent health care profession, Florence Nightingale's accomplishments were far broader and equally significant. Her use of statistics seems to be the true beginning of evidence-based medicine and health care, only now, 150 years later, becoming the new paradigm in medicine. Nightingale's innovative work in statistics began with her insistence on the importance of gathering data and went on to include the design of data-gathering tools and methods of data analysis and presentation. Her data were unassailable and her graphics were persuasive. Many of the reforms she advocated, both within the British Army and in civilian affairs, were realized in her lifetime. Within a year of her return from the Crimea, the Secretary of State for War issued an order to organize what became the Statistical Branch of the Army Medical Department. Other of her reforms, such as her advocacy of a university chair in statistics, came later. Her work in statistics was recognized by the profession in 1858, when she was elected the first woman Fellow of the Royal Statistical Society.[9]

RKS

[ 91

ENDNOTES

1. Cook, vol. 1, p. 428, chapter title.

2. Cook, quoted in vol. 1, p. 100.

3. Marion Diamond and Mervyn Stone. "Nightingale on Quetelet." *Journal of the Royal Statistical Society*, A vol. 144, part 1 (1981), pp. 66–79.

4. Cook, quoted in vol. 1, p. 324.

5. Great Britain. *Report of the Commissioners Appointed to Inquire into the Regulations affecting the Sanitary Condition of the Army*. . . . (cat. no. 83).

6. *Report of the Proceedings of the Fourth Session of the International Statistical Congress*. London: Printed by George Edward Eyre and William Spottiswoode, 1861, pp. 181–183.

7. Nelson and Rafferty, pp. 126–127.

8. Lynn McDonald, ed. *Collected Works of Florence Nightingale*. 16 vols. Waterloo, Ontario: Wilfrid Laurier University Press, 2002–2012.

9. http://www.rss.org.uk/site/cms/contentCategoryView.asp?category=42 (accessed September 7, 2012).

REFERENCES

Cohen, I. Bernard. "Florence Nightingale." *Scientific American*, vol. 250, no. 3 (March 1984), pp. 128–137.

Cook, Edward. *The Life of Florence Nightingale*. 2 vols. London: Macmillan & Co., 1913.

McDonald, Lynn. *Florence Nightingale at First Hand*. Waterloo, Ontario: Wilfrid Laurier University Press, 2010.

Nelson, Sioban and Anne Marie Rafferty, eds. *Notes on Nightingale: The Influence and Legacy of a Nursing Icon*. Ithaca: Cornell University Press, 2010.

ITEMS EXHIBITED

83. Florence Nightingale. "Answers to Written Questions addressed to Miss Nightingale by the Commissioners." In *Report of the Commissioners Appointed to Inquire into the Regulations Affecting the Sanitary Condition of the Army, the Organization of Military Hospitals, and the Treatment of the Sick and Wounded; with Evidence and Appendix*. Pp. 361–394 and ten charts. London: Printed by George Edward Eyre and William Spottiswoode, 1858. Original printed blue wrapper. [SEE FIG. 14]

This huge document is the report of the Royal Commission created by Queen Victoria at the instigation of Florence Nightingale – "I wish we had her at the War Office." Nightingale's innovations began with an insistence on data gathering and went on to the design of data-gathering tools and methods of data presentation, in today's terms, evidence-based health care. The ten charts in the report include examples of her "coxcomb" diagrams to illustrate that most of the deaths in the Crimean War were due to preventable causes, not bullets.

Nightingale developed some of her concepts from the work of the social statistician

Adolphe Quetelet. Her colleague Dr. William Farr prepared the charts. Many of her reforms were realized because she had friends in high places in the British government.

84. Florence Nightingale. *A Contribution to the Sanitary History of the British Army during the Late War with Russia*. London: John W. Parker and Son, 1859. (Courtesy, The New York Academy of Medicine Library.)

This report, attributed to Nightingale, contains three of her diagrams. The color chart documenting " . . . Causes of Mortality in the Army in the East" divides the causes of death into three categories: battle wounds; fever, cholera, diarrhea, dysentery, and scurvy; and ordinary diseases. The area of the wedges represents the mortalities. "Mitigable and preventible pestilences" were the cause of most deaths.

# MARIE MEURDRAC 1610?–1680

## BIOGRAPHY

Marie Meurdrac, the author of an early treatise on practical chemistry, was one of two girls born into an aristocratic French family in north-central France. While her older sister took pleasure in riding and hunting, Marie, more serious, involved herself in community life, serving as godmother to several village children. Records indicate that in 1625 she married Henri de Vibrac, commander of Charles de Valois's guard unit, and that she lived in the château of Grosbois.

Except for Meurdrac's friendship with the Countess de Guiche, a woman of illustrious lineage who welcomed her into the château – and to whom Meurdrac would later dedicate her treatise – little is known about Meurdrac's life. The historian Jean-Pierre Poirier suggests that Meurdrac was not satisfied simply overseeing the management of the chateau.[1] The widowed countess, similarly restless, recognized a kindred spirit in Meurdrac and became her benefactress, supporting her decision to dedicate herself to the study of chemistry and its benefits for the women in the community. Meurdrac and the countess endeavored to improve the lives of less fortunate women.

Self-taught, Meurdrac began by reading contemporary pharmaceutical works, and she was especially inspired by the work of the chemist Nicolas Lémery (1645–1715). Apparently she performed a large number of chemical experiments, and the results provided the source material for her chemistry book, *La Chymie Charitable et Facile, en Faveur des Dames* (1666),[2] with subsequent French editions in 1674, 1680, 1687, and 1711. Her treatise proved to be popular and it appeared in six German editions and one Italian edition.[3]

Meurdrac's book, written for the common reader, is organized around six topics: chemical operations and apparatus; materials derived from plants; products derived from animals; inorganic chemistry; substances useful in medicine; and products for women's beauty and health. Meurdrac's book is very much a contemporary chemistry text, invoking the three Paracelsian principles – mercury, the spirit; sulfur, the soul; and salt, the body – as essential qualities. Although containing no recognized discoveries, the book clearly demonstrates her knowledge and competence as a practical chemist and an apothecary.

In the lengthy foreword, Meurdrac candidly reveals her hesitation about publishing the treatise that had been intended solely as a permanent record of her research. Further, she questions the larger issue of a woman's right to publish and its ensuing consequences. "I remained irresolute in this inner struggle for two years," she writes. "I objected to myself that it was not the profession of a lady to teach, that she should remain silent, listen and learn, without displaying her own knowledge . . . that a reputation gained thereby is not ordinarily to her advantage since men always scorn and blame the products of a woman's mind." Meurdrac ultimately decided to go public as Damoiselle [sic] M.M., declaring that "minds have no sex and that if the minds of women were cultivated like those of men and if enough time and expense were spent to instruct them, they would be equal to those of men.[4]

Her decision to publish was rooted in her unwavering belief that her practical book was useful in remedying women's illnesses as well as a guide to the preservation of their health. Unquestionably an early feminist who broke ground in an area where few women dared to tread, Meurdrac felt that not sharing knowledge that could ameliorate the lives of others would be a betrayal of the Catholic principle of charity as well as incompatible with her inquisitive temperament. A true seventeenth-century *femme savante*, Meurdrac along with other learned women, who were later ridiculed in Molière's comedy *Les Femmes Savantes* (1672), would not be deterred in the quest to investigate, comprehend, and contribute to the advancement of scholarship.

## SIGNIFICANT CONTRIBUTIONS

In the seventeenth century, chemistry was an uncommon topic for a book written for the common reader and especially for a book written by a woman. Marie Meurdrac's text is one of practical chemistry, in which she argues that other chemistry books lead mostly to speculation and that doing chemistry is more instructive than contemplating it.[5] A recent commentary on Meurdrac's work highlights her understanding that a primary aspect of chemistry is the separation and isolation of substances from "Mixts" and that she doubted, probably correctly from her practical experience, that soluble compounds of gold and silver could be created as claimed by other chemists.[6]

Meurdrac's book appeared in twelve European editions, and except for the first French edition, her text had a publisher, thus suggesting that her book was of continuing value. Twenty-five percent of her book is devoted to topics of special interest to women. One can perhaps attribute the birth of modern cosmetology to her work with perfumes, bleaches, face and hand creams, hair dyes, and skin cleansers, and with formulas for the treatment of itching and diseases of the skin. Notwithstanding the emphasis on chemistry applied to women's special needs, the majority of the text is devoted to significant topics in general chemistry.

PR AND RKS

## ENDNOTES

1. Poirier, p. 171.

2. The date 1656 on the title page of a few copies is apparently the result of a typesetting error. The *privilège* and *approbation* dates in Stanford University's 1656-dated copy are December 20, 1665 and December 10, 1665, the same dates as in copies dated 1666 on the title page. In addition, one can observe that the title page in 1666-dated copies is a cancel leaf, that is, an inserted single leaf presumably to replace the title page with the incorrect date.

3. Tossi, p. 81, fn. 13.

4. Marie Meurdrac. *La Chymie Charitable et Facile, En Faveur des Dames. Par Damoiselle M.M.* Nouvelle edition présentée et annotée par Jean Jacques. Paris, 1999. Foreword, pp. 16–18. Translated from the French by Paulette Rose.

5. Meurdrac (1999), p. 31.

6. Tossi, pp. 74 and 77.

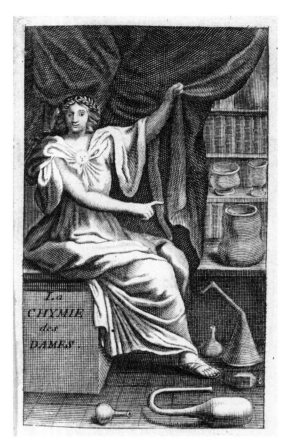

Fig. 15. Engraved title page of the Paris 1687 edition of Marie Meurdrac's *La Chymie Charitable et Facile, en Faveur des Dames*. (Courtesy, The Othmer Library of Chemical History, The Chemical Heritage Foundation.) [CAT. 86]

## REFERENCES

Bishop, Lloyd O. and Will S. DeLoach. "Marie Meurdrac – First Lady of Chemistry?" *Journal of Chemical Education*, vol. 47, no. 6 (June 1970), pp. 448–449.

Poirier, Jean-Pierre. "Marie Meurdrac (Madame de Vibrac)." In *Histoire des Femmes de Science en France du Moyen Age à la Révolution*. Paris: Éditions Pygmalion, Gérard Watelet, 2002, pp. 170–176.

Tossi, Lucia. "Marie Meurdrac: Paracelsian Chemist and Feminist." *Ambix*, vol. 48, part 2 (July 2001), pp. 69–82.

## ITEMS EXHIBITED

85. M[arie] M[eurdrac]. *La Chymie Charitable et Facile, en Faveur des Dames*. Paris: Rue des Billettes et Rue du Plastre, 1666. (Courtesy, The Othmer Library of Chemical History, The Chemical Heritage Foundation.)

In the seventeenth century, chemistry was an uncommon topic for a book by a woman and for the common reader. Meurdrac's book is devoted to practical chemistry, and she argues that doing experiments is more instructive than contemplating speculative hypotheses, the subject of most chemistry books of the period. The book treats six topics derived from the author's experiments: chemical operations, plant-based substances, animal-based products, inorganic chemistry, medicinal substances, and products for women's beauty and health.

In the foreword to her book, Meurdrac reveals that her treatise was originally intended solely as a record of her research and that she was hesitant about publishing it. She also remarks that with study women can be the equal of men.

86. [Marie Meurdrac]. *La Chymie Charitable et Facile, en Faveur des Dames*. 3rd ed. Paris: Laurent d'Houry, 1687. (Courtesy, The Othmer Library of Chemical History, The Chemical Heritage Foundation.) [SEE FIG. 15]

Presumably a manifestation of its value, Meurdrac's chemistry text was often and widely reprinted. Known are five French and six German editions and one Italian edition. This "Troisième edition" – actually the fourth as there were Paris 1674 and Lyon 1680 imprints after the first edition of 1666 – includes an engraved title page and a folding plate of chemical symbols.

87. M[arie] M[eurdrac]. *La Chymie Charitable et Facile, en Faveur des Dames*. Paris: Rue des Billettes, 1656. Facsimile title page with presumed typesetting error. (Courtesy, Department of Special Collections, Stanford Libraries.)

A few copies of Meurdrac's book are known with a 1656 date on the title page. Apparently never noticed previously is that the printed date "1656" must be a typesetting error. The *privilège* and *approbation* dates in a 1656-dated copy examined are December 20, 1665 and December 10, 1665, the same dates as in copies with "1666" on the title page. Further examinations revealed that the title page in two 1666-dated copies is a cancel leaf, that is, a single inserted leaf, presumably to replace the original title page with the misprinted date. Thus, statements in bibliographies and other references for the first appearance of Meurdrac's text in 1656 are spurious.

# MARIE-GENEVIÈVE-CHARLOTTE THIROUX D'ARCONVILLE 1720–1805

## BIOGRAPHY

Marie-Geneviève-Charlotte Thiroux d'Arconville, born in Paris, stands out as a woman who made her mark in the sciences as a chemist and in the world of letters as a biographer, novelist, essayist, historian, and translator. The daughter of a wealthy farmer-general, she married at age fourteen Louis-Lazare Thiroux d'Arconville, also a farmer-general and later a president in the *Parlement* of Paris. The eldest of their three sons, Louis Thiroux de Crosne, was lieutenant-general of the Paris police during the Jean Calas affair. He was guillotined during the Reign of Terror and his mother was imprisoned for several months.

Thiroux d'Arconville's life took a turn at twenty-two when she contracted smallpox, leaving her badly blemished. Renouncing an active social life, she dedicated herself to scholarly pursuits. A Jansenist and a philanthropist, she founded a hospice near her country home in Meudon. Above all, she was practical and understood the hurdles faced by women who dared to enter fields dominated by men. Accordingly, all of her fifty-some publications appeared with the garb of anonymity to avoid gender bias in the reception of her work.

The restraints on female education did not prevent Thiroux d'Arconville from learning English and Italian while also frequenting the King's Garden in Paris, where lectures in physics, anatomy, botany, and chemistry were open to the public. She spent her days reading and writing in Paris, where she had access to the King's library, and in her country home, where she had a laboratory for experiments. Although she avoided Parisian society, she opened her home to such distinguished men of letters as Voltaire, Denis Diderot, and Lamoignon de Malesherbes, as well as to the botanist Bernard de Jussieu and the eminent chemists Antoine-Laurent Lavoisier, Antoine Fourcroy, and Pierre-Joseph Maquer.

She was particularly drawn to chemistry and began to work under the tutelage of Macquer, who asked her to translate Peter Shaw's *Chemical Lectures* (1731), which was published as *Leçons de Chymie Propres à Perfectionner la Physique, le Commerce et les Arts* (1759). She appended to the work a ninety-four-page introduction with a comprehensive account of the history of applied chemistry. In her technical writings, she did not hesitate to correct perceived errors of other scientists, such as Shaw.

Continuing to guard her anonymity, Thiroux d'Arconville prepared for publication *Traité d'Ostéologie* (1759), a translation of Alexander Monro's *Anatomy of the Human Bones* (1729). She enhanced Monro's treatise, which is not illustrated, by introducing thirty-one plates depicting skeletons and bones. The illustrations were initially and mistakenly attributed to Jean J. Süe, a professor of anatomy under whose auspices the work was published.

Over a ten-year period beginning in 1754, Thiroux d'Arconville performed experiments on the decomposition of organic substances. The result was her book *Essai Pour Servir à l'Histoire de la Putréfaction* (1766). On the title page, she signed this original work "Par le Traducteur des Leçons de Chymie de M. Shaw." A pioneer in a new field of study – putrefaction – she focused her research on the effectiveness of methods to preserve meat. She carried out 317 experiments, recording observations about the conditions and the results.

The range of subject matter in Thiroux d'Arconville's oeuvre is astonishing. Most of her writings, including translations of scientific papers published in London, were collected and published in seven volumes.[1] They include two of her best-known essays, *Sur l'Amitié* (1761) and *Des Passions* (1764); her numerous translations of English and Italian novels, including those of George Lyttleton and Aphra Behn; and biographies of such historical figures as King Francis II and Queen Marie de Medici.

A contemporary review of Thiroux d'Arconville's treatise on putrefaction captured the distinct personality of this brilliant eighteenth-century woman.[2] The reviewer underscored the importance of the work and praised the depth of knowledge demonstrated in both medicine and chemistry, calling it the product of a "highly distinguished physician." Beseeching the author, presumed to be a man, to reveal his identity, the reviewer concluded that the writer was more interested in being a helpful citizen than in furthering a brilliant reputation. Such was the modest, dedicated, and prolific Thiroux d'Arconville.

## SIGNIFICANT CONTRIBUTIONS

It was not until the early nineteenth century when modern ideas about food preservation appeared. So it would seem that the experiments and ideas of Marie-Geneviève-Charlotte Thiroux d'Arconville in the eighteenth century were innovative. Her experiments were mostly original and her book is possibly the first monograph on the subject of putrefaction and how to minimize it. The almost 600-page text is organized into a series of experiments, with the date and the weather conditions stated and observations recorded. A discussion section follows the description of each series of experiments. A summary of the research results is presented in the form of tables on ten large folding leaves.

All the while – before, during, and after the period of her chemical research – Thiroux d'Arconville was having published all manner of literature, essays, and scientific translations. Only a few of her works are easy to find today, and her collected works in seven volumes is uncommon. Volume three of the seven-volume work contains most of her scientific translations except for the two books discussed here.

PR AND RKS

## ENDNOTES

1. [M.-G.-C. Thiroux d'Arconville]. *Mêlanges de Litterature, de Morale et de Physique.* 7 vols. Amsterdam: aux Dépens de la Compagnie, 1775–1776.

2. "Essai Pour Servir à l'Histoire de la Putréfaction. Par le Traducteur des Leçons de Chymie de M. Shaw." *Journal des Sçavans, pour l'année MDCCLXVI* (October, 1766), pp. 683–687.

## REFERENCES

Bret, Patrice. "Arconville, Marie-Geneviève Charlotte Thiroux d'." In *New Dictionary of Scientific Biography*, vol. 1. Detroit: Charles Scribner's Sons/Thomson Gale, 2008, pp. 91–93.

Poirier, Jean-Pierre. "Marie Genèvieve Charlotte Thiroux d'Arconville." In *Histoire des Femmes de Science en France du Moyen Age à la Révolution*. Paris: Éditions Pygmalion, Gérard Watelet, 2002, pp. 265–270.

Schiebinger, Lorna. *The Mind Has No Sex? Women in the Origins of Modern Science.* Cambridge: Harvard University Press, 1991.

88. Pierre Shaw. *Leçons de Chymie Propres à Perfectionner la Physique, le Commerce et les Arts*. Paris: Jean Thomas Herissant, 1759. [M.-G.-C. Thiroux d'Arconville], translator and author of the introduction.

Thiroux d'Arconville was encouraged by the chemist P.-J. Macquer to translate Peter Shaw's very popular *Chemical Lectures* into French. She is identified as the translator in a 1768 letter from Macquer to a colleague. The translation was probably done from the second edition (1755) of Shaw's book. To the translation, Thiroux d'Arconville added notes and a ninety-four-page preliminary discourse that provides a comprehensive history of applied chemistry.

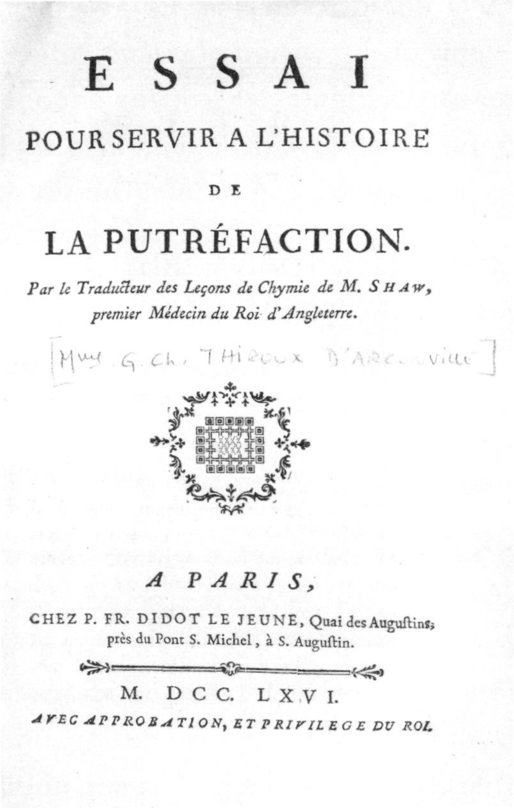

ESSAI

POUR SERVIR A L'HISTOIRE

DE

LA PUTRÉFACTION.

*Par le Traducteur des Leçons de Chymie de M. SHAW, premier Médecin du Roi d'Angleterre.*

A PARIS,

CHEZ P. FR. DIDOT LE JEUNE, Quai des Auguſtins, près du Pont S. Michel, à S. Auguſtin.

M. DCC. LXVI.

AVEC APPROBATION, ET PRIVILEGE DU ROI.

Fig. 16. Title page of Thiroux d'Arconville's 600-page text describing her experiments on putrefaction. [CAT. 89]

89. [M.-G.-C. Thiroux d'Arconville]. *Essai Pour Servir à l'Histoire de la Putréfaction*. Paris: Didot le Jeune, 1766. [SEE FIG. 16]

Over a ten-year period, Thiroux d'Arconville performed 317 original experiments on the decomposition of organic substances. The result was this 600-page text, possibly the first on the subject. She identified herself on the title page only as the translator of Shaw's chemistry book. The volume is organized into a series of observations with the date and weather conditions stated and her observations described. A summary of the research is presented in the form of tables on ten large folding plates. The book was highly praised in a contemporary review published in the *Journal des Sçavans*.

90. [Marie-Geneviève Thiroux d'Arconville]. *Des Passions*. Par l'Auteur du Traité de l'Amitié. Londres [i.e., Paris], 1764.

In addition to her scientific works, Thiroux d'Arconville published numerous essays, none of which she signed in her own name. They were often attributed to Diderot, whom she befriended. Here, she defines passion as any sentiment carried to its extreme and further reduces her definition to "love" and "ambition." These two principal passions with all their nuances are studied in both men and women. The engraved title page vignette and two additional plates illustrate the full trajectory of irrational behavior.

# ELIZABETH FULHAME  fl. 1780–1794

## BIOGRAPHY

What little is known about this author of an experimental chemistry book is found in the preface of the book[1] and in a few research notes about another English chemist.[2] Elizabeth Fulhame is believed to have been the wife of Dr. Thomas Fulhame, who graduated M.D. at Edinburgh University in 1784 and who remained there engaged in chemistry until about 1790. When he became the husband of Elizabeth Fulhame is unknown. Nor is any other information about her known.

In the eleven-page preface to her text, Mrs. Fulhame wrote that in 1780 she conceived the idea of using chemical reactions to make metallic cloths, by which she meant silk material with embedded metal. Although initially discouraged by her husband, she began experiments that yielded some success, but it was not until the early 1790s, she reported, that she was able to produce pieces of cloth embedded with gold and silver deposited by chemical reactions, in some cases aided by light.

Unfavorable judgments by friends, she wrote, continued to inhibit her to try to publish her work until October 1793, when "a celebrated philosopher" saw her work, approved it, and offered to have a paper presented to the Royal Society of London. The celebrated philosopher was probably the famous English, and later American, chemist Joseph Priestley, who did mention meeting her in London.[3] With this approbation, her mind was made up, and she was now eager to publish her work to prevent a "prowling plagiary" from stealing her ideas. She understood that her experiments on calcination, that is oxidation, of metals were equivalent to combustion, and so she adopted *An Essay on Combustion* as the main title of her book.

In the preface, she has more to say about the contents of her book, in particular that it is not a simple narrative of her experiments, but rather is organized so that that the observations suggest general principles and ideas for future work. Later in the preface, she devotes text to the matters of people uninterested in learning and of women involved with learning, and comments that "some are so ignorant, . . . and are chilled with horror at the sight of learning, in whatever shape it may appear; and should the spectre appear in the shape of a woman, the pangs, which they suffer, are truly dismal."[4] She concluded the preface with a statement truly representative of the scientific method, to wit, that she has offered her opinion of what her experiments demonstrate, but that she is "willing to relinquish it, as soon as a more rational appears."[5]

## SIGNIFICANT CONTRIBUTIONS

Until recently, Mrs. Fulhame's book had been noticed by only a few writers. J. F. Coindet, the Swiss physician who discovered iodine therapy for goiter, praised the book in a long review in 1798.[6] In the same year, Benjamin Thompson referred to the "ingenious and lively Mrs. Fulhame" as the inspiration for his experiments about the effect of light on chemical reactions.[7] More recently, historians of photography have noted that Mrs. Fulhame described experiments about the effect of light on chemical reactions with silver compounds and that metallic silver was created in a way similar to that in photographic processing. It was suggested that Mrs. Fulhame was creating printed images with light-induced chemical reactions and that she should be considered, therefore, a key person in the history – or perhaps pre-history – of photography.[8]

What is clear from her text is that she had a recognizably modern conception of chemical reactions, such as oxidation and reduction, and that she had observed and described the concept of catalysis, the idea that certain chemicals can participate in and aid a chemical reaction without themselves being consumed. Her observations of catalytic reactions were described in detail in 1903.[9] Modern physical chemists have also noted her descriptions of catalysis.[10] Today, catalysis is essential for the production of most chemical products.

Mrs. Fulhame took the unusual position for the period that neither the chemistry of the Phlogistians, for example Joseph Priestley, nor that of the Anti-Phlogistians, Lavoisier and his followers, explained adequately her observations, but she seems to have favored the latter, which at least puts her on the correct side of history. The concluding section of her book is significant for expressing an understanding of aspects of the reciprocal nature of oxidation and reduction and for presenting the concept of the steady-state condition in natural processes.

RKS

## ENDNOTES

1. Mrs. Fulhame. *An Essay on Combustion, . . .*, London, 1794 (cat. no. 91).

2. T. S. Wheeler and J. R. Partington. *The Life and Work of William Higgins, Chemist (1763–1825)*. New York: Pergamon Press, 1960, fn. 139, pp. 121–122.

3. Joseph Priestley. *The Doctrine of Phlogiston Established, and that of the Composition of Water Refuted*. 2nd ed. Northumberland, PA: printed for P. Byrne by Andrew Kennedy, 1803. p. 80.

4. Mrs. Fulhame, London, 1794, p. xi.

5. Mrs. Fulhame, London, 1794, p. xiii.

6. J. F. Coindet. "De l'ouvrage de Mme. Fulhame, intitulé: . . ." *Annales de Chimie*, vol. 26 (April 19, 1798), pp. 58–85.

7. Benjamin Count of Rumford (Benjamin Thompson). "An Inquiry concerning the Chemical Properties that have been attributed to Light." *Philosophical Transactions of the Royal Society,* vol. 88 (1798), pp. 449–468.

8. Larry Schaaf. *Out of the Shadows – Herschel, Talbot, & the Invention of Photography*. New Haven: Yale University Press, 1992, pp. 23–25.

9. J. W. Mellor. "History of the Water Problem (Mrs. Fulhame's Theory of Catalysis)." *Journal of Physical Chemistry*, vol. 7, no. 8 (November 1903), pp. 557–567.

10. Keith J. Laidler. *The World of Physical Chemistry*. Oxford: Oxford University Press, 1993, pp. 250, 277–278.

## REFERENCES

Davenport, Derek A. "Fulhame, Elizabeth." *Oxford Dictionary of National Biography*, vol. 21. Oxford: Oxford University Press, 2004, pp. 128–129.

Davenport, Derek A. and Kathleen M. Ireland. "The Ingenious, Lively and Celebrated Mrs. Fulhame and the Dyer's Hand." *Bulletin for the History of Chemistry*, no. 5 (Winter 1989), pp. 37–42.

## ITEMS EXHIBITED

91. Mrs. Fulhame. *An Essay on Combustion, with a View to a New Art of Dying and Painting.* London: printed for the author, 1794. (Courtesy, The Othmer Library of Chemical History, The Chemical Heritage Foundation.) [SEE FIG. 17]

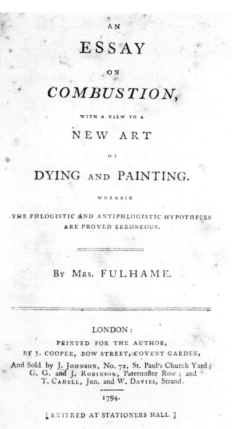

Fig. 17. Title page from the London edition of Fulhame's report on her experiments in chemistry. (Courtesy, The Othmer Library of Chemical History, The Chemical Heritage Foundation.) [CAT. 91]

In her only publication, Elizabeth Fulhame described her research to find a process to produce metal-embedded silk fabrics. The text is not a simple narrative of the experiments, but rather is organized to suggest general principles as she understood the results. Among her prescient observations were catalytic reactions and light-induced chemical reactions, and she had a recognizably modern conception of oxidation and reduction reactions.

Based upon her experiences of being discouraged by others, Mrs. Fulhame commented in the preface about people uninterested in learning and notes that "some are so ignorant, . . . and chilled with horror at the sight of learning, . . . and should the spectre appear in the shape of a woman, the pangs, which they suffer, are truly dismal."

92. Mrs. Fulhame. *An Essay on Combustion, with a View to a New Art of Dying and Painting.* Philadelphia: James Humphreys, 1810. (Courtesy, The Othmer Library of Chemical History, The Chemical Heritage Foundation.)

Mrs. Fulhame's text was reprinted in Philadelphia, and also in a German translation in 1798. The British, and later American, chemist Joseph Priestley was the person who in late 1793 encouraged her to publish her research. With Priestley's approbation, her mind was made up, and she became eager to publish her experiments to prevent a "prowling plagiary" from stealing her ideas. "Combustion" in the modern sense is not the subject of her book, but remarkably she used the term in the title to refer, correctly, to oxidation processes.

# DOROTHY CROWFOOT HODGKIN 1910–1994

## BIOGRAPHY

A Nobel scientist and peace activist, Dorothy Mary Crowfoot was born in Cairo, Egypt, where her father was engaged in archaeological and educational projects. She and her three sisters grew up mostly in England in the absence of their parents. Later, while an undergraduate, she assumed responsibility for her three younger sisters while their parents continued to live in Khartoum and travel throughout the Middle East. Dorothy believed that her experiences in the absence of her parents accounted for her independent, self-reliant attitude.[1]

Dorothy Crowfoot began the study of crystal structures as an undergraduate at Oxford University, England. Upon graduation she was accepted into the premier research group in crystallography at Cambridge University. She developed a life-long commitment to structural biochemistry, the determination of the crystal structure of biochemically important materials. She was among the first to obtain x-ray diffraction photographs of protein crystals. Although it was not possible at the time to extract crystal structures from such patterns, her experiments indicated that structural determinations would eventually be possible. While still a graduate student, she developed rheumatoid arthritis, which although severe, did not impede her activities.

Prior to completion of the Ph.D. in 1937, Dorothy Crowfoot received a fellowship at Somerville College, Oxford, and the remainder of her professional life was spent there. Also in that same year, she married Thomas Hodgkin, but only later did she begin using the name Hodgkin on publications. Marriage, including three children, did not deflect her from her career path.

Hodgkin was able to choose scientific problems considered difficult or unsolvable at the time, but problems that she believed she could tackle successfully. She is credited as the primary person responsible for the determination of the molecular structure of three important biological substances – penicillin, vitamin B12, and insulin. Upon the solution of penicillin in 1945, a colleague commented "you will get the Nobel Prize for this," but upon Hodgkin's comment that she would rather be elected a Fellow of the Royal Society, he replied "that's more difficult."[2] Hodgkin did, in fact, become an F.R.S. in 1945, the third woman to be elected. More honors followed. She received the unshared Nobel Prize in Chemistry in 1964, and, after Florence Nightingale, Hodgkin was only the second woman to receive Great Britain's highest civilian honor, the Order of Merit.

Hodgkin's husband came from a Quaker family and her mother had a strongly altruistic character; these factors may have influenced Dorothy Hodgkin to become deeply associated with anti-war organizations. Many of these organizations had Communist Party members, thus perhaps explaining why she was refused a visa to enter the United States for a few years. Her visa applications were not helped by her reception of the award of the Lenin Peace Prize. She organized Pugwash Conferences and was president of the Pugwash organization for many years. Dorothy campaigned against the Vietnam War and worked to send aid to Hanoi. Her meeting with General Jaruzelski in Warsaw at the same time that the Polish government was violently suppressing a Solidarity demonstration was controversial even within the Pugwash organization.

Hodgkin's successes can, in part, be traced to the network of researchers in which she found herself as a student: both her Ph.D. professor, J. D. Bernal, and his Ph.D. professor, W. H. Bragg, had large research groups with women in the majority. It is also the curious case, for which various explanations have been offered, that the field of crystallography has been more attractive generally to women than many other scientific fields. Hodgkin created her own network of research collaborators from among her colleagues. She had many research students, about half of whom were women. She actively supported her students in conflict with the university rule that women lost their fellowships and stipends upon marriage, and she was able to have the rule overturned on an individual basis.[3] Hodgkin herself never believed that her gender had been an obstacle to her advancement.[4] The obituary in *The* (London) *Times* provides this description of her character: ". . . a woman with no enemies, a woman of infinite understanding, compassion, simplicity and an enduring serenity."[5]

## SIGNIFICANT CONTRIBUTIONS

What distinguished Dorothy Crowfoot Hodgkin from her contemporaries in crystallography was the skill and determination to extend the methods of x-ray diffraction to substances far more complex than had been attempted before. She recognized that crystal structures could be solved in the absence of knowing the exact chemical formula of materials. She was the pioneer in the development of methods for complete three-dimensional solutions of crystal structures. Of great consequence was the determination of the chemical formula and structure of penicillin during World War II; this research was kept secret because of its military significance and published in 1949.[6] Her work with penicillin demonstrated the significance of this type of research, as it led to the development of many other antibiotics.

Hodgkin's second great achievement, in 1956, was the determination of the chemical formula and structure of vitamin B12, the substance in raw liver that was used to treat pernicious anemia.[7] This work was done at Oxford University with a team that included her students and researchers and a collaborator in the United States. Her third great technical accomplishment was the solution, in 1969, of the structure of insulin[8] – thirty-four years after having taken her first x-ray diffraction image of the substance. Dorothy Crowfoot Hodgkin's work in crystallography not only solved important contemporary problems but also led to the methods of analysis used extensively today for the study of complex biochemical materials.

RKS

## ENDNOTES

1. Ferry, p. 14.

2. Quoted in Ferry, p. 214.

3. Jenny P. Glusker. "Dorothy Crowfoot Hodgkin (1910–1994)." *Protein Science*, vol. 3, no. 12 (December 1994), p. 2468.

4. Ferry, pp. 2, 247.

5. *The Times*. London, July 30, 1994. http://www.physics.ucla.edu/~cwp/dev/hodgkObit.html (accessed August 27, 2012).

6. D. Crowfoot, et al. "The X-ray Crystallographic Investigation of the Structure of Penicillin" (cat. no. 94).

7. Dorothy Crowfoot Hodgkin, et al. "The Structure of Vitamin B12. I. . . . ," (cat. no. 95).

8. Margaret Joan Adams, et al. "Structure of Rhombohedral 2-Zinc Insulin Crystals." *Nature*, vol. 224, no. 5218 (November 1, 1969), pp. 491–495.

## REFERENCES

Ferry, Georgina. *Dorothy Hodgkin: A Life.* London: Granta, 1998.

Glusker, Jenny P. "Dorothy Crowfoot Hodgkin (1910–1994)." In *Out of the Shadows*, edited by Nina Byers and Gary Williams. Cambridge: Cambridge University Press, 2006, pp. 240–261.

Hunter, Graeme K. "Hodgkin, Dorothy Mary Crowfoot." In *New Dictionary of Scientific Biography*, vol. 3. Detroit: Charles Scribner's Sons/Thomson Gale, 2008, pp. 333–339.

Julian, Maureen M. "Women in Crystallography." In *Women of Science – Righting the Record*, edited by G. Kass-Simon and Patricia Farnes. Bloomington and Indianapolis: Indiana University Press, 1993, pp. 335–383.

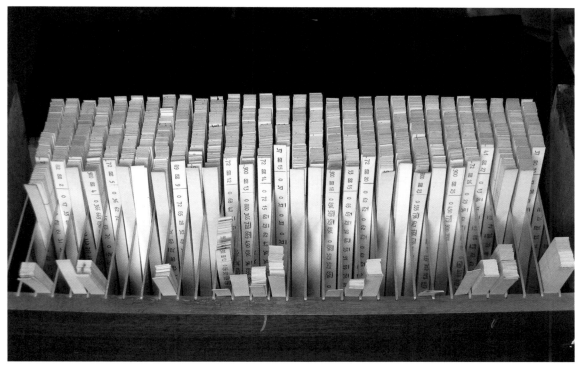

Fig. 18. A pre-electronic calculating device, Beevers-Lipson strips, of the type used by Dorothy Hodgkin in her early work in crystallography; one box of set of two. (Courtesy, Jenny P. Glusker.) [CAT. 98]

## ITEMS EXHIBITED

93. Dorothy Crowfoot Hodgkin. Photograph, Philadelphia, 1970. (Courtesy, Jenny P. Glusker.)

94. D. Crowfoot, et al. "The X-ray Crystallographic Investigation of the Structure of Penicillin." In *The Chemistry of Penicillin*, edited by Hans T. Clarke, et al., pp. 310–367. Princeton: Princeton University Press, 1949.

Extensive research on penicillin began during World War II. Dorothy Hodgkin led a team that determined its crystal structure in the absence of knowing in advance the detailed chemical composition and then used the resulting information to deduce the composition. The work reported in this publication – important for the development of antibiotics – was released from military security classification as of January 1, 1946.

95. Dorothy Crowfoot Hodgkin, et al. "The Structure of Vitamin B12. I. An Outline of the Crystallographic Investigation of Vitamin B12." *Proceedings of the Royal Society* A vol. 242, no. 1229, pp. 228–263 (October 29, 1957). Issue in wrapper.

The crystal structure of vitamin B12 – the substance in raw liver used to treat pernicious anemia – was described in a series of six papers by Dorothy Hodgkin and her team of students and colleagues. They also demonstrated that the chemical composition, not directly obtainable by chemical analysis, could be determined from the crystallographic information. The journal departed from its usual printing in black and white and illustrated the articles not only in color but with overlays in color. Parts II to VI appeared in subsequent issues of the *Proceedings*.

96. Dorothy Crowfoot Hodgkin. "Vitamin B12." *Proceedings of the Royal Institution of Great Britain*, vol. 42, part VI, no. 199, pp. 377–396 (1969). Issue in wrapper.

In this invited review, Hodgkin notes that her work with vitamin B12 began in 1948. As she was reluctant to publish prematurely, her first significant publication was delayed until 1955. In that year, a Cambridge chemist, later a 1957 Nobel awardee, took information from her paper, added some minor chemical information, and presented a paper that was interpreted by the press as the announcement of the structure of vitamin B12. Shortly thereafter, a letter appeared in the press giving Hodgkin and her colleagues the "main credit."

97. Dorothy Crowfoot Hodgkin. "Insulin, Its Chemistry and Biochemistry." The Bakerian Lecture, 1972. *Proceedings of the Royal Society*, A vol. 338, no. 1614, pp. 251–275 (June 28, 1974). Bound volume.

After the structure determinations of penicillin and vitamin B12, Hodgkin's third technical accomplishment – this one after her 1964 Nobel Prize in Chemistry – was the solution, in 1969, of the structure of insulin, thirty-four years after having taken her first x-ray diffraction image of the substance. This later review paper is based on her presentation in an endowed lecture series that began in 1775. She continued work with insulin and her last paper on the subject appeared in 1988.

98. Beevers-Lipson strips, one box of set of two. (Courtesy, Jenny P. Glusker.) [SEE FIG. 18]

Until the mid-1930s, the determination of complex crystal structures from x-ray diffraction data could require many days of trial-and-error computations. The invention of

Beevers-Lipson strips significantly reduced computation times. Thousands of strips of paper printed with an indexing scheme and intermediate trigonometric solutions are organized in two boxes. Based upon x-ray diffraction data, strips are selected using the indexing scheme, laid out in proper order on a table, and the numbers on the strips summed to calculate coefficients of a mathematical solution, which is a possible electron-density map.

In her Nobel lecture, Dorothy Hodgkin mentioned how important Beevers-Lipson strips were for her early work. This set of Beevers-Lipson strips is borrowed from one of Hodgkin's Ph.D. students from the vitamin B12 research project.

99. Dorothy Crowfoot Hodgkin. T.L.S. to Linus C. Pauling, April 1982. (Courtesy, Special Collections and Archives Research Center, Oregon State University.)

Late in her life, Dorothy Hodgkin was active in anti-war organizations, including as president of the Pugwash organization. The 1982 Pugwash meeting was scheduled to be held in Warsaw shortly after martial law had been declared in Poland, and attendance became a very controversial topic, especially among the American delegates. In this letter Hodgkin solicits Linus Pauling to sign a declaration against the growing threat of nuclear weapons. Hodgkin created much further controversy by meeting with General Jaruzelski while she was in Warsaw.

# ROSALIND E. FRANKLIN 1920–1958

## BIOGRAPHY

Born into a family of merchant bankers in London, Rosalind Franklin, even when young, was not inclined to accept what she was told without evidence. About the existence of God, she asked "Well, anyhow, how do you know He isn't a She?"[1] Unlike most young women, she chose to be a scientist. With an outstanding education in science and mathematics, she began in 1938 at Cambridge, where during her second year she discovered the subject of crystallography.

Faced with the decision to continue at Cambridge for a Ph.D. or to possibly be called up for military service, she chose instead a position with the British Coal Utilisation Research Association (BCURA), where she participated in research about carbonaceous materials such as coal and charcoal. At BCURA, she displayed her penchant to want to do things herself by using, without training, machine tools in the mechanical shop. Her work yielded a Ph.D. thesis in 1945 and her first two important publications.[2]

In early 1947, Franklin relocated to a research facility in Paris and found much to like about Paris and her French acquaintances, but family relationships and a three-year fellowship at King's College, London drew her back to England in early 1951. The first intimation of conflict came about when she discovered that women were not permitted to take their lunch in the King's senior common room. She was not happy to discover that her research assignment had been changed, without her being asked, to crystallographic studies of nucleic acids (DNA). Major conflicts later arose because of ambiguity about her position relative to that of another researcher Maurice Wilkins and because Wilkins tried to create a collaborative atmosphere that was undesired by Franklin.

Early in her research at King's College, Franklin made key discoveries: initially about how to prepare DNA specimens to obtain sharp x-ray diffraction patterns and later that DNA can exist in two types, called A and B, depending upon the water content.[3] Having obtained good diffraction patterns of both types, Franklin made what a later close friend and colleague, Aaron Klug, called a "misjudgment" in selecting type A to try to analyze.[4] She reasoned that type A could be solved by an analytical crystallographic approach, whereas type B seemed impossible except perhaps by building models, a method of work she generally rejected. During this period, James Watson and Francis Crick at Cambridge began building hypothesized helical models of DNA.

Without Franklin's knowledge, Watson was shown her now famous diffraction pattern, so-called Photograph 51, of type-B DNA by Wilkins and given parameters from the data. In his autobiography, Wilkins states that he was given this photograph by Franklin's student, Raymond Gosling, and was told by Gosling that Franklin had authorized the use of the photograph for any purpose.[5] The interpretation of the photograph was so obvious to Watson that the next day he began ordering components to build a model, and six days later Watson and Crick began building their now-famous structure. Additional information was obtained from a contract report written by Franklin and shown to Watson, in all innocence, by a colleague. Watson and Crick saw and understood the information that Franklin had obtained months earlier but had not recognized for all its implications.

Very unhappy at King's College, Franklin wrote "I'm abandoning an unfinished job . . . to get out of King's without further delay."[6] At Birkbeck College, in late 1953 she began research on the tobacco mosaic virus (TMV), a model for viruses in general. Here again she found herself not on good terms with some staff members, but as a research team leader she had the full support of the director, J. D. Bernal. Within about two years, Franklin was recognized as an authority on the TMV.[7] During the period 1955 to 1958, her research yielded important publications, the last of which was submitted under the name (The Late) R. E. Franklin.

## SIGNIFICANT CONTRIBUTIONS

In her short life, Rosalind Franklin achieved the status of an authority in the three research topics she undertook. The work with carbonaceous substances led her to discover molecular sieve behavior in materials, now of industrial importance. More significantly, she distinguished graphitic carbon and vitreous (glassy) carbon, each with uniquely different properties and both important.[8] Her development of x-ray diffraction methods applicable to carbonaceous materials was the ideal background for the later work with DNA and the TMV.

Her discoveries of a new specimen preparation method and that water content was significant for the structure of DNA were essential to obtain unambiguous x-ray diffraction data. Unknowingly, however, her data provided the critical information to Watson and Crick, who had the background to recognize key aspects of the DNA structure from the diffraction pattern. Franklin's scientific style – analytical and data-driven rather than intuitive and model-driven – may well have played a role in the DNA story. Notwithstanding that final credit went to others, it remains that two generally unhappy years in a new field of research brought her very close to the "secret of life."

Upon moving to Birkbeck College, Franklin applied her skill with x-ray diffraction to the tobacco mosaic virus, with the objective to understand how it infects a host cell. In 1954, Watson had demonstrated the helical structure of the TMV, but did no further research on its structural details. Franklin, in addition to the determination of the geometry of the major sub-units around the helix, located the TMV's infective element, its ribose nucleic acid, RNA.

Conflict and unpleasantness are found at various times during Rosalind Franklin's career. In many cases the difficulties were clashes of personality and of style of doing scientific work, not gender issues. Her tendency to resist the collaborative process common in scientific work may have been a factor. By the time of her early death at the age of thirty-seven, she had made significant contributions in every subject she touched.

RKS

## ENDNOTES

1. Quoted in Glynn, p. 12.

2. Rosalind E. Franklin, in *Transactions of the Faraday Society* (cat. no. 101).

3. Rosalind E. Franklin and R. G. Gosling. "The Structure of Sodium Thymonucleate Fibres. I. The Influence of Water Content." *Acta Crystallographica*, vol. 6, no. 8–9 (September 10,1953), pp. 673–677.

4. Aaron Klug. "The Discovery of the DNA Double Helix." *Journal of Molecular Biology*, vol. 335, no. 1 (January 2, 2004), p. 12.

5. Maurice Wilkins. *The Third Man of the Double Helix*. Oxford: Oxford University Press, 2003, pp. 197–198.

6. Quoted in Maddox. p. 205.

7. Angela N. H. Creager and Gregory J. Morgan. "After the Double Helix: Rosalind Franklin's Research on Tobacco Mosaic Virus." *Isis*, vol. 99, no. 2 (June 2008), pp. 239–272.

8. Peter J. Harris. "Rosalind Franklin's Work on Coal, Carbon, and Graphite." *Interdisciplinary Science Reviews*, vol. 26, no. 3 (2001), pp. 204–210.

## REFERENCES

Glynn, Jenifer. "Rosalind Franklin: 50 Years On." *Notes & Records of the Royal Society,* vol. 62, no. 2 (June 20, 2008), pp. 253–255.

Glynn, Jenifer. *My Sister Rosalind Franklin*. Oxford: Oxford University Press, 2012.

Klug, Aaron. "Franklin, Rosalind Elsie." *Oxford Dictionary of National Biography*, vol. 20. Oxford: Oxford University Press, 2004, pp. 795–797.

Maddox, Brenda. *Rosalind Franklin – The Dark Lady of DNA*. New York: HarperCollins, 2002.

Olby, Robert. *The Path to the Double Helix*. Seattle: University of Washington Press, 1974.

Watson, James D. *The Annotated and Illustrated Double Helix*. Ed. by Alexander Gann and Jan Witkowski. New York: Simon & Schuster, 2012.

## ITEMS EXHIBITED

100. Rosalind Franklin. Photograph. Undated. [SEE FIG. 19]

101. Rosalind E. Franklin. "A Study of the Fine Structure of Carbonaceous Solids by Measurements of True and Apparent Densities. Part I. Coals," pp. 274–286. With ". . . Part II. Carbonized Coals," pp. 668–682. In *Transactions of the Faraday Society*, vol. 45 (1949). Bound volume.

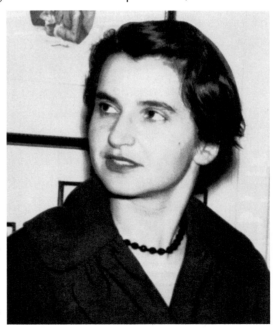

Fig. 19. Portrait, undated, of Rosalind Franklin. [CAT. 100]

Franklin's first research work, and the subject of her Ph.D. thesis, focused on various types of carbon. Although she did not study diamond (pure carbon), Franklin made key discoveries about graphitic and vitreous carbon, each with uniquely different and useful properties. Her development of x-ray diffraction methods applicable to carbonaceous materials was the ideal background for her later work. These two papers are her earliest significant publications.

102. Rosalind E. Franklin and R. G. Gosling. "Molecular Configuration in Sodium Thymonucleate." *Nature,* vol. 171, no. 4356, pp. 740–741 (April 25, 1953). Issue in wrapper.

In the issue of *Nature* with the famous paper by Watson and Crick proposing the structure of deoxyribonucleic acid (DNA), Franklin and her student published a diffraction pattern of DNA and discussed its implications for the structure of DNA, concluding that "our general ideas are not inconsistent with the model proposed by Watson and Crick in the preceding communication." Franklin, however, was not able to propose structural details, which Watson and Crick learned in the process of model-building.

Nowhere in the paper by Watson and Crick is it noted that Watson had been shown, without Franklin's knowledge, one of her diffraction patterns. Acknowledged only is that they were aware of the "general nature of unpublished experimental results and ideas of . . . Dr. R. E. Franklin . . . "

103. Rosalind E. Franklin, A. Klug, and K. C. Holmes. "X-ray Diffraction Studies of the Structure and Morphology of Tobacco Mosaic Virus." In *The Nature of Viruses,* edited by G. E. W. Wolstenholme and Elaine C. P. Millar, pp. 39–55. London: J. & A. Churchill, 1957.

By 1955 Franklin was recognized as an authority on the tobacco mosaic virus (TMV), a model for virus studies in general. She had determined the basic geometry of the huge molecule and located the infective element, its ribose nucleic acid (RNA). This review paper is based upon her invited presentation at a symposium. Her last publication appeared just a year after this collection of conference papers, under the name (The Late) R. E. Franklin.

104. Rosalind Franklin. A.L.S. to Colin Franklin, Paris, October 5, 1950. (Courtesy, Colin Franklin.)

In this letter, written to her brother during one of her dark moods, Franklin describes her regrets in leaving Paris to take a position in the research group with Maurice Wilkins at King's College, London. She predicts being unhappy at King's, which turned out to be accurate. It was here that she did the crystallographic research with DNA.

# MARIA CUNITZ 1610–1664

BIOGRAPHY[1,2]

A woman about whom little is known, but who wrote the "earliest surviving scientific work by a woman on the highest technical level of its age,"[3] Maria Cunitz (Kunicia, Cunitia, Kunic) grew up in Wołów (Wohlau), in the western part of Poland. Her parents were from distinguished Silesian families, and by 1615 the family was living in Šwidnica (Schweidnitz). Documented tradition presents a picture of intelligence and accomplished learning in the sciences, languages, and the arts when she was still a child. In 1630 Cunitz married Elias von Löven (Kreczmar), a physician who shared her interest in astronomy and had published on the subject. They had three sons.

Maria Cunitz and her husband, as Protestants caught in the midst of the Counter-Reformation and the Thirty Years' War, moved westward to Byczyna (Pitschen) about 1630. Her three siblings, instead, converted to the Catholic religion. A few years later Maria Cunitz and her husband retired, temporarily, to a quiet village under the protection of a convent near Lubnice, and it was here that she did the mathematical work and the writing for her book *Urania Propitia*, which was a complete reworking of Johannes Kepler's *Tabulae Rudolphinae* (the *Rudolphine Tables*, named after Emperor Rudolph II of Bohemia) of 1627.

Her book, self-published, appeared in 1650, and must have been a severe challenge to the typesetter. Among more than 550 pages are found almost 300 pages of tables of numbers with as many as 1000 numbers on one page and with a variety of layouts of the tables, sometimes on one page. The descriptive text, in about 250 pages, appears in both Latin and German and contains a variety of small tables integrated within the text on many pages. In the four-page "Maritus ad Lectorem" (Husband to the Reader), her husband states that she is the sole author of the book. *Urania Propitia* was dedicated to the Holy Roman Emperor Ferdinand III, and Cunitz's handwritten letter to Ferdinand III asking permission to publish the book survives.[4]

A major fire in Byczyna on May 25, 1656 destroyed the Cunitz house, which presumably accounts for the paucity of her papers and manuscripts. About the time her book appeared, Cunitz began correspondence with numerous astronomers, including Johannes Hevelius, the doyen of contemporary astronomers, in Danzig. Known surviving documents are mostly letters, which remain an unexplored source of possibly new information, to correspondents in Paris and Vienna.

## SIGNIFICANT CONTRIBUTIONS

Astronomy was the most advanced and mathematically complex science during the seventeenth century. It had two primary applications: determination of the ecclesiastical calendar and prognostication from astrological information based upon the position of the planets. In 1627 Johannes Kepler had published *Tabulae Rudolphinae*, a book filled with mathematics and tables of numbers to calculate the positions of the planets at any time in the past or future. Kepler's book was based upon his discovery of the three laws that mathematically define the orbits of the planets around the sun. Books with the contents copied from Kepler's *Tabulae Rudolphinae* began to appear in 1639.

Maria Cunitz's *Urania Propitia*, however, is a totally original work. Her objective was to reduce the complexity of the calculations found in Kepler's book. A key modification was to eliminate calculations with logarithms. Her book provided all new tables and new calculation methods to simplify obtaining solutions to problems of planetary motion. A modern scholar has estimated that one solution from Kepler's tables requires at least one hour of computation time with numerous chances for errors to be introduced, and he provided a detailed analysis demonstrating the merits of the tables and procedures developed by Cunitz.[5] Considering the mathematical accomplishment represented by Maria Cunitz's book, one is led to conclude that she was probably the most advanced scholar in mathematical astronomy of her time.

RKS

## ENDNOTES

1. http://muzeum-kupiectwa.pl/index.php?page=zycie-dzielo-astronom-marii-kunic-cunitii-1610-1664 (accessed August 6, 2012). Web site for exhibition, Muzeum Dawnego Kupiectwa w Świdnicy, October–December 2008.

2. *Astronom Maria Kunic (Cunitia) 1610–1664*. Świdnica: Muzeum Dawnego Kupiectwa w Świdnicy, 2008. Exhibition catalog.

3. Swerdlow, p. 81.

4. Ingrid Guentherodt. "Maria Cunitia. Urania propitia: Intendiertes, erwartetes und tatsächliches Lesepublikum einer Astronomin des 17. Jahrhunderts." *Daphnis*, vol. 20, no. 2, (1991), pp. 311–353. Illustration p. 346.

5. Swerdlow, pp. 93–117.

REFERENCES

Hatch, Robert Alan. "Cunitz [Cunitia, Cunitiae], Maria." In *Biographical Encyclopedia of Astronomers*, edited by Thomas Hockey. New York: Springer, 2007, pp. 263–264.

Swerdlow, Noel M. "Urania Propitia, Tabulae Rudophinae faciles redditae a Maria Cunitia Beneficent Urania, the Adaption of the Rudolphine Tables by Maria Cunitz." In *A Master of Science History, Essays in Honor of Charles Coulston Gillispie*, edited by Jed Z. Buchwald. Heidelberg: Springer, 2012, pp. 81–121.

ITEMS EXHIBITED

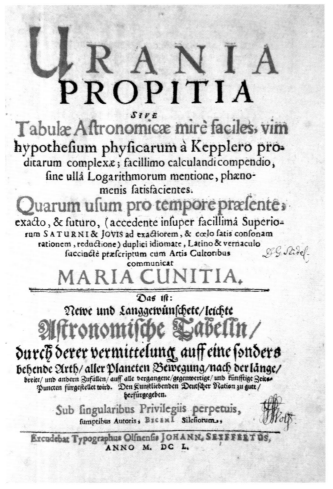

Fig. 20. Title page of Maria Cunitz's 550-page book, *Urania Propitia*, of astronomical calculations. (Courtesy, Owen Gingerich.) [CAT. 106]

105. Statue of Maria Cunitz. Photograph, Świdnica, 2009. Stanislaw Strzyzynski, sculptor. (Courtesy, Dr. Radoslaw Skowron, Museum Dawnego Kupiectwa Świdnicy.)

Maria Cunitz lived in Świdnica (Schweidnitz), Poland from about 1615 until 1630, at which time she married and moved westward with her husband to escape the ravages of the Thirty Years' War. The depiction is purely the artist's idea.

106. Maria Cunitia. *Urania Propitia*. Olesnica (Oels): Johann Seyffert, for the author, 1650. (Courtesy, Linda Hall Library.) [SEE FIG. 20]

Maria Cunitz's 550-page book is a complete reworking of the mathematics of Johannes Kepler's *Rudolphine Tables* (1627) for the computation of planetary positions. Her objective was to simplify the calculations, primarily by elimination of logarithms. Her book provides 300 pages of tables of numbers and a new calculation method glossed with 250 pages of text written in both German and Latin. Considering the mathematical accomplishment represented by her book, Cunitz seems to have been the most advanced scholar in mathematical astronomy of her time.

116 ]

# CECILIA H. PAYNE-GAPOSCHKIN  1900–1979

## BIOGRAPHY

Cecilia Helena Payne – perhaps qualified to be considered the founder of modern astrophysics – grew up in England within a family of almost all women, including three generations of aunts. Her traditional early education reveals itself by the literary allusions in her later writings. With a scholarship to Newnham College in 1919, Cecilia Payne began studies in physics at Cambridge University, where opportunities to attend lectures by England's leading physicists and astronomers presented itself. Upon discovering that Newnham College had an observatory with a damaged telescope, she repaired its mechanical parts and began using it.

Near the end of her college days, Payne came to suspect that the only future for her in England was as a teacher. A. J. Comrie, a recent Cambridge Ph.D. in astronomy, suggested to her that opportunities for women in astronomy might be better in the United States, and after a lecture he introduced Payne to Harlow Shapley, director of the Harvard College Observatory. Almost immediately upon being introduced, Payne asked Shapley if she could come to Harvard to study astronomy. A few months later, in the fall of 1923, she began life as a graduate student in Cambridge, MA.

Harvard did not have a graduate program in astronomy, and it was suggested that she become a degree candidate in the Department of Physics. That idea fell through because the Department of Physics refused to accept a woman candidate for a Ph.D. As a result, Shapley essentially created a graduate school of astronomy with Payne as the first and only student. As there had been no graduate department in astronomy, there were no graduate courses, and for her degree Payne only had to write a thesis. Just two years after her arrival at Harvard, she had already published six papers and had completed, as Otto Struve, one of the most distinguished astronomers of the twentieth century, stated, "undoubtedly the most brilliant Ph.D. thesis[1] ever written in astronomy."[2] Payne's thesis research had a key role in the development of astrophysics.

Cecilia Payne's later research subjects included the peculiarities of highly luminous stars and of stars whose brightness varies with time. Notwithstanding that she taught graduate courses and was the advisor for Ph.D. research students, for many years she was regarded only as a technical assistant to Shapley. She commented: "I was paid so little that I was ashamed to admit it to my relations in England."[3] After the department had grown, Shapley attempted to get Payne a permanent position, but reported that he was rebuffed by Harvard's president. Not until 1956 was she appointed a professor at Harvard, and at the same time she was made chairperson of the Department of Astronomy – the first woman at Harvard to be appointed a department chair. She continued research work at Harvard almost to the end of her life.

In Germany in 1933 Cecilia Payne had met a Russian astronomer Sergei Gaposchkin, who was stateless and seeking a way to escape the Nazi regime. Upon her return to the United States, she arranged for a visa and for a position at Harvard for him. In early 1944 they were married. The Gaposchkins had three children. Much of Payne's later research work was done jointly with her husband.

## SIGNIFICANT CONTRIBUTIONS

Whether or not Otto Struve's statement about Cecilia Payne's thesis remains valid more than fifty years later, the fact remains that her thesis results completely upset the contemporary wisdom concerning the chemical composition of the universe in suggesting that stars are all basically composed of the same elements and are mostly hydrogen and helium. Her conclusion that the light elements dominate the composition of the stars was considered wrong at the time, and in response to a comment – "clearly impossible" – in a letter from her thesis advisor, Henry Norris Russell at Princeton,[4] she felt forced to write in her thesis that the data about hydrogen

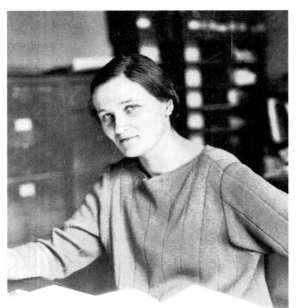

Fig. 21. Cecilia Payne at Harvard College Observatory, ca. 1928. (Courtesy, Smithsonian Institution Archives. Image 2009-1326.) [CAT. 107]

and helium were "spurious" and "almost certainly not real."[5] However, her conclusion that the two lightest elements dominate the composition of the stars was generally accepted within just a few years. Russell was the first to confirm her conjecture and has been cited often for the discovery. A recent paper points out that in 1925 no astronomer would have accepted the claim of a graduate student, male or female, for the universe being so "profoundly different than previously supposed."[6] The discovery that the light elements dominate stellar compositions was the first milestone in the development of the theoretical understanding of the nuclear reactions from which stars derive their energy.

Payne's thesis was also a milestone for the recognition that the physics of the atom is the basis for understanding the physics of the universe. She applied the contemporary quantum theory of atomic structure to the problem of the chemical composition of the stars and made the startling discovery that the large variety of light-emission spectra among stars was not due to variation of the chemical composition but to physical conditions such as temperature. She went on to identify a method to calculate the relative abundance of many elements in stellar atmospheres.

Cecilia Payne's later research work on highly luminous stars and on variable stars also made important contributions to understanding the physics of the universe. Notwithstanding her accomplishments, when the president of Princeton University asked Henry Norris Russell to suggest a candidate for a professorship, he replied, referring to Payne, that the best candidate in America "alas, is a woman!"[7]

RKS

## ENDNOTES

1. Cecilia H. Payne. *Stellar Atmospheres* (cat. no. 109).

2. Otto Struve and Velta Zebergs. *Astronomy of the 20th Century*. New York: Macmillan, 1962, p. 220.

3. Haramundanis, p. 221.

4. Henry Norris Russell to Cecilia H. Payne. Typescript carbon copy of letter, January 14, 1925, p. 3 (Princeton University, Henry Norris Russell Papers).

5. Payne, *Stellar Atmospheres*, pp. 186 and 188.

6. David H. DeVorkin. "Extraordinary Claims Require Extraordinary Evidence: C. H. Payne, H. N. Russell and Standards of Evidence in Early Quantitative Stellar Spectroscopy." *Journal of Astronomical History and Heritage*, vol. 13, no. 2 (July 2010), p. 139.

7. David H. DeVorkin. *Henry Norris Russell: Dean of American Astronomers*. Princeton: Princeton University Press, 2000, p. 341.

## REFERENCES

Gingerich, Owen. "Payne-Gaposchkin, Cecilia Helena." In *New Dictionary of Scientific Biography*, vol. 6. Detroit: Charles Scribner's Sons/Thomson Gale, 2008, pp. 49–52.

Haramundanis, Katherine, ed. *Cecilia Payne-Gaposchkin*. Cambridge: Cambridge University Press, 1996. Autobiography of Cecilia Payne-Gaposchkin edited by her daughter.

Lankford, John and Rickey L. Slavings. "Gender and Science: Women in American Astronomy, 1859–1940." *Physics Today*, vol. 43, no. 3 (March 1990), pp. 58–65. Also, letters in response in *Physics Today*, vol. 43, no. 8 (August 1990), pp. 91–92.

Rubin, Vera C. "Cecilia Payne-Gaposchkin (1900–1979)." In *Out of the Shadows*, edited by Nina Byers and Gary Williams. Cambridge: Cambridge University Press, 2006, pp. 158–168.

107. Cecilia Payne. Photograph. Cambridge, MA, Harvard College Observatory, ca. 1928. (Courtesy, Smithsonian Institution Archives. Image 2009-1326.) [SEE FIG. 21]

108. Cecilia H. Payne. "Astrophysical Data Bearing on the Relative Abundance of the Elements." *Proceedings of the National Academy of Sciences*, vol. 11, no. 3, pp. 192–198 (March 1925). Offprint.

Well before completing her Ph.D. thesis, Payne had published numerous papers with some of her results. In this article she presented some of her conclusions about the relative abundances of the elements in the stars. She felt compelled to question her own conclusions about the concentration of hydrogen and helium in the stars, as they differed so much from contemporary ideas.

109. Cecilia H. Payne. *Stellar Atmospheres*. Harvard Observatory Monographs, No. 1. Cambridge, MA: Harvard Observatory, 1925. Ph.D. thesis.

Payne's Ph.D. research played a key role in the development of astrophysics. Her work demonstrated that the physics of the atom is the basis for understanding the physics of the stars, and she was the first to apply the new quantum theory of atomic structure to astrophysical problems. Her discovery that the light elements hydrogen and helium dominate stellar compositions was the first milestone to understanding the nuclear reactions from which stars derive their energy.

Payne's thesis results about stellar composition were not believed at the time. To have her thesis accepted, she had to carefully weaken her claims on pages 186 and 188. However, her data are in the thesis, thus establishing her priority, which however went unnoticed until much later.

110. Cecilia Payne-Gaposchkin. *Introduction to Astronomy*. Englewood Cliffs, NJ: Prentice-Hall, 1954.

Payne-Gaposchkin's introductory textbook was written, in part, to emphasize that astronomy "played no small part in the cultural development of the human race." Making use of her traditional education, she included literary and historical allusions to astronomy, quoting, for example, Goethe, Edna St. Vincent Millay, Shakespeare, Pindar, Dante, Tennyson, Walt Whitman, and others at each chapter. Her book was the first introductory text to put emphasis on the physics of the stars and stellar systems.

# AUGUSTA ADA BYRON  Countess of Lovelace, 1815–1852

## BIOGRAPHY

Augusta Ada Byron was the child of Lord Byron. Just weeks after her birth, Ada's mother announced that she wanted a separation, which she achieved by threatening to expose Byron's alleged incestuous relationship with his half-sister and Ada's namesake, Augusta Leigh. Ada's childhood was beset by illnesses, including more than three years as a semi-paralyzed invalid. Her mother, although perhaps not a model of motherhood, provided Ada with a good education. She began mathematical studies at age five and continued them for twenty years, first with Mary Somerville, translator of a French text on mathematical astronomy, and then with Augustus De Morgan, a preeminent analytical mathematician and logician. In addition to formal studies, Ada's mother arranged meetings to introduce Ada to prominent members of the scientific community in London.

In 1833 Ada met Charles Babbage, the inventor of mechanical computing concepts and machines, and by 1836 she had become fascinated by Babbage's first calculating device, the Difference Engine. Babbage, in the meantime, had turned his attention to his second calculator, the Analytical Engine, and Ada – recently married to William King, later Earl of Lovelace – engaged with Babbage about his ongoing work.

In the fall of 1841, after eight years of work, Babbage described his landmark Analytical Engine at a seminar in Turin. Although the Engine was never constructed, there is no doubt that in conception and design, it embodied all of the essential elements of what is recognized today as a general-purpose digital computer. L. F. Menabrea, an Italian military engineer who attended the seminar, reported the presentation the following year in an obscure Swiss serial, and Babbage urged Ada Lovelace to translate the report into English. In fact, Lovelace undertook a far larger task: adding to her

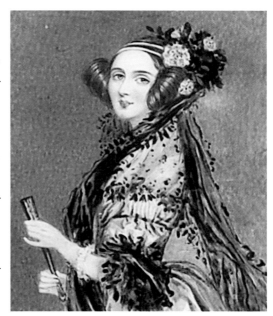

Fig. 22. Victorian watercolor portrait of Ada Lady Lovelace by Edward Taylor. (Courtesy, H. M. Fletcher and Nigel Phillips.) [CAT. 111]

translation a series of important explanatory "Notes" substantially longer than Menabrea's article. The result, published in 1843, was a two-part, sixty-six-page paper,[1] generally considered "the most important paper in the history of digital computing before modern times."[2] Lovelace's writing was clear, powerful, and to the point. And at times the Notes showed her literary heritage: "We may say most aptly that the Analytical Engine weaves algebraical patterns just as the Jacquard-loom weaves flowers and leaves."[3] But she did not simply clarify how the Analytical Engine worked – although she certainly did that; she gave us remarkable insights into the significance and implications of its workings.

There is repeated foreshadowing of Turing, Shannon, and von Neumann – the twentieth-century giants in computing – in her work, often with no evidence that the thoughts originated with Babbage. Indeed, the extent of Babbage's own appreciation of Lovelace's insight is reflected in one of his letters, commenting on her draft notes: "I am very reluctant to return your admirable & philosophic Note A. Pray do not alter it . . . All this was impossible for you to know by intuition and the more I read your notes the more surprised I am at them and regret not having earlier explored so rich a vein of the noblest metal."[4]

Honoring the contemporaneous conventions of her class and her gender, Lady Lovelace signed the "Notes" simply with her initials, A.A.L., creating an instant mystery. The first published explanation came five years later, when the translation and notes were ascribed to "a lady of distinguished rank and talent," with a footnote identifying her as "Lady Lovelace."[5]

After her work with Babbage, Lovelace suffered continuing bouts of severe illnesses, both mental and physical, until her death at age thirty-six of complications from uterine cancer. Her "Notes" were rediscovered and reprinted almost exactly a hundred years later, bringing a well-deserved, posthumous recognition. As an acknowledgment of the contributions of Ada Lovelace to computing, the trademark "Ada" was registered in 1979 for a U.S. Department of Defense computer language.

SIGNIFICANT CONTRIBUTIONS

The Menabrea-Lovelace paper is the most important documentation of the capability and power of Babbage's Analytical Engine. Ada Lovelace's deep conceptual understanding of Babbage's device and how it operated is set out in a clearly written and farsighted description of the Analytical Engine. Her description makes it clear that Babbage's machine is the conceptual forerunner of modern digital computing.

In her "Notes " Lovelace stated in particular that the Engine could not "originate any thing," only do "whatever we know how to order it to perform."[6] She pointed out the critical importance of conditional branching – the Engine could make decisions by comparing numbers – and the reuse of code; the significance of the Engine's conceptual ability to perform operations with symbols as well as numbers; and the difference between what was possible to compute and what was simply impracticable. As an example of operations with symbols that do not represent a quantity, she suggested that "the engine might compose . . . music of any degree of complexity . . . "[7] And she included an example by converting an "algebraic working out" provided by Babbage – correcting what Babbage later acknowledged to have been "a grave mistake"[8] – into a detailed series of steps – a nineteenth-century "computer program" – showing precisely how his Engine could perform a complex calculation.

PJM AND RKS

## ENDNOTES

1. [Ada Lady Lovelace]. "Notes by the Translator," pp. 691-731. With: L. F. Menabrea. "Sketch of the Analytical Engine invented by Charles Babbage, Esq." (cat. no. 112).

2. Alan G. Bromley, introduction to *Babbage's Calculating Engines: A Collection of Papers*. [Edited] *by Henry Prevost Babbage*. Cambridge: MIT Press, 1984, p. xv.

3. [Ada Lady Lovelace]. "Notes by the Translator," p. 696.

4. Quoted in Toole, p. 197.

5. Charles Richard Weld. A *History of the Royal Society*, vol. 2. London: J. W. Parker, 1848, p. 387.

6. [Ada Lady Lovelace]. "Notes by the Translator," p. 722.

7. Ibid., p. 694.

8. Charles Babbage. *Passages from the Life of a Philosopher*, p. 136. London: Longman, Green, Longman, Roberts, & Green, 1864, p. 136.

## REFERENCES

Fuegi, John and Jo Francis. "Lovelace & Babbage and the Creation of the 1843 'Notes.'" *IEEE Annals of the History of Computing*, vol. 25, no. 4 (October–December 2003), pp. 16–26.

Grier, David A. "King, Ada Augusta, Countess of Lovelace." In *New Dictionary of Scientific Biography*, vol. 4. Detroit: Charles Scribner's Sons/Thomson Gale, 2008, pp. 118–120.

Stein, Dorothy. *Ada: A Life and Legacy*. Cambridge: MIT Press, 1987.

Toole, Betty Alexandra. *Ada, the Enchantress of Numbers*. Mill Valley, CA: Strawberry Press, 1992. A selection of her letters.

111. Ada Lady Lovelace. Watercolor portrait by Edward Tayler, Victorian period. (Courtesy, H. M. Fletcher and Nigel Phillips.) [SEE FIG. 22]

112. [Ada Lady Lovelace]. "Notes by the Translator," pp. 691–731. [With:] L. F. Menabrea. "Sketch of the Analytical Engine invented by Charles Babbage, Esq." Translated by Ada Lady Lovelace, pp. 666–690. In *Scientific Memoirs, Selected from the Transactions of Foreign Academies of Science and Learned Societies, and from Foreign Journals*, vol. III, edited by Richard Taylor. London: Printed by Richard and John E. Taylor, 1843.

The Menabrea-Lovelace papers are the most important documentation of the capabilities of Charles Babbage's Analytical Engine, the nineteenth-century conceptual forerunner of a general-purpose computer. Ada Lovelace's understanding of Babbage's machine and how it operated are set out in a clearly written and farsighted description.

In her *Notes*, Lovelace stated that the Engine could not "originate any thing," only do "whatever we know how to order it to perform." She pointed out, among other features, that the Engine itself could make decisions. As an example of operations with symbols, she suggested that "the engine might compose . . . music . . . " And she included a numerical application, the calculation of Bernoulli numbers, by creating a detailed series of steps – a nineteenth-century "computer program" – showing how Babbage's Engine could perform a complex calculation.

# GRACE MURRAY HOPPER 1906–1992

## BIOGRAPHY

From a profoundly different culture and separated by one hundred years from Augusta Ada Byron, Countess of Lovelace,[1] whose conceptual ideas about how a computer could perform were remarkably prescient, Grace Murray Hopper was probably the single most important person in the early development of programming languages for modern digital computers.

Grace Brewster Murray was born in New York in 1906, into a family with military traditions and to an independent mother with a love of mathematics. From an early age, Grace Murray demonstrated curiosity and fascination with things mechanical combined with a natural talent for mathematics. She was an undergraduate at Vassar, and from there went to Yale to enter the Ph.D. program in the mathematics department. About this time, she married Vincent Foster Hopper, but the marriage did not last, although Grace kept the name Hopper. In 1934 she received the Ph.D. in mathematics from Yale. Hopper was an associate professor of mathematics at Vassar during World War II when she took a leave of absence to join the Navy WAVES.

After graduating first in her Midshipman's School class, she received a commission and was assigned to the Bureau of Ships Computation Project at Harvard University. When Hopper arrived at the Computation Laboratory in July 1944, the Automatic Sequence Controlled Calculator, the Harvard Mark I, had just become operational under the leadership of Howard Aiken. As she later recalled, the famously brusque Aiken greeted her with, "Where the hell have you been?"[2] and – pointing to the 50-foot-long, 35-ton, electro-mechanical relay calculator – told her that she had one week to learn "how to program the beast and to get a program running."[3] Hopper quickly mastered the new machine and became its chief programmer.

Interest in the Mark I led to the publication of a 561-page operations manual, the first of its kind and a landmark publication.[4] A noted historian of computing described its significance this way: "The Manual is one of the first places where sequences of arithmetic operations for the solution of numerical problems by machine were explicitly spelled out. It is furthermore the first extended analysis of what is now known as computer programming since Charles Babbage's and Lady Lovelace's writings a century earlier. The instruction sequences, which one finds scattered throughout this volume, are thus among the earliest examples anywhere of digital computer programs."[5] Although Hopper was the principal author of the *Manual*, as even a cursory reading of the preface makes clear and as has been noted elsewhere,[6] authorship was attributed simply to "The Staff of the Computation Laboratory." She did receive credit, but as the second-listed co-author, when a condensed version of the *Manual* appeared later.[7]

After the war, Hopper turned down a full professorship at Vassar and stayed at Harvard as a Navy researcher working on new computers. In 1949 she joined the small group at the fledgling Eckert-Mauchly Computer Corporation developing the UNIVAC I, the first large-scale, commercial, electronic digital computer.

Based on the time consuming and frustrating experience of "programming" the Harvard computers, Hopper believed that programming, not hardware, would be the key bottleneck for the future of computing. She set out to address this problem by creating a program that used the computer itself to translate, i.e., "compile," instructions written in a high-level language – a "source language" that could be understood and used by people who were not computer specialists – into "machine language" instructions that the computer could implement. Hopper termed this program "A-o," for automatic programming language zero – the first compiler. Hopper explained this work in her milestone article, "The Education of a Computer."[8] In it she talks of using the UNIVAC to take on "the dull labor of writing and checking programs" so that "the programmer may return to being a mathematician." Hopper concludes by writing: "Thus by considering the professional programmer (not the mathematician), as an integral part of the computer, it is evident that the memory of the programmer and all information and data to which he can refer is available to the computer subject only to translation into suitable language. . . . UNIVAC at present has a well grounded mathematical education fully equivalent to that of a college sophomore, and it does not forget and does not make mistakes. It is hoped that its undergraduate course will be completed shortly and it will be accepted as a candidate for a graduate degree."[9]

Hopper's team went on to the development of mathematical languages that were predecessors of FORTRAN. And she led the development of the "B-o" language, FLOW-MATIC, designed to compile instructions for use in commercial and business applications. With Hopper's urging, technical skill, and proselytizing, this language became the basis of the ubiquitous "Common Business Oriented Language," COBOL – still in use throughout the world and on virtually every computing platform more than 50 years after its creation. In short, Hopper was probably the single most important person in the early history of programming languages.

After her work at the Eckert-Mauchly Computer Corporation, Hopper had leadership positions with other computer manufacturers. She kept her Naval Reserve status until 1967, when she reached the mandatory retirement age. A few months after her retirement from the Reserves, she was recalled to active duty, and during the next nineteen years she rose through the ranks to rear admiral. At the Pentagon, her initial assignment was to standardize the programming languages used by the Navy. The standards became mandatory throughout the Department of Defense and subsequently in the computer industry. Although Grace Hopper was "an admiral who never went to sea,"[10] in 1997 the USS *Hopper* was commissioned.

SIGNIFICANT CONTRIBUTIONS

Only a select few could be claimed to have had an impact matching that of Grace Hopper in the development of modern digital computing. Of greatest importance was her very early recognition that programming, not hardware, would be

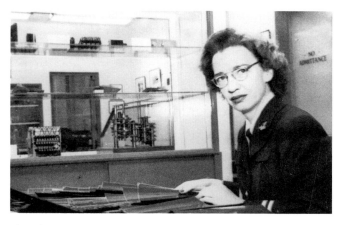

Fig. 23. Navy Lieutenant Grace Hopper in the Harvard Computation Laboratory, 1947. (Courtesy, Grace Murray Hopper Collection, Archives Center, National Museum of American History, Smithsonian Institution.) [CAT. 113]

the limitation to the future of computing technology. To solve this problem, she developed the concept of a compiler, a computer program that would translate an easy-to-learn computer language into a machine language that the computer could implement. Hopper had distinguished careers, both in the Navy – as a flag-rank officer – and in the commercial computing industry. Her work created fundamental programming standards that remain valid today.

PJM AND RKS

## ENDNOTES

1. See section on Augusta Ada Byron, Countess of Lovelace in this publication.

2. Grace Hopper. "Commander Aiken and My Favorite Computer." In *Makin Numbers: Howard Aiken and the Computer*, edited by I. Bernard Cohen and Gregory W. Welch. Cambridge: MIT Press, 1999, p. 185.

3. Williams, *Grace Hopper: Admiral of the Cyber Sea*, p. 26.

4. The Staff of the Computation Laboratory. *A Manual of Operation for the Automatic Sequence Controlled Calculator* (cat. no. 114).

5. Paul E. Ceruzzi. In *A Manual of Operation for the Automatic Sequence Controlled Calculator*. CBI Reprint Series for the History of Computing, vol. 8. Cambridge: MIT Press, 1985, p. xvii.

6. I. Bernard Cohen. *Howard Aiken: Portrait of a Computer Pioneer*. Cambridge: MIT Press, 1999, p. 163.

7. Howard H. Aiken, and Grace M. Hopper, "The Automatic Sequence Controlled Calculator" (cat. no. 115).

8. Grace Murray Hopper. "The Education of a Computer" (cat. no. 116).

9. Ibid., p. 249.

10. Williams "Hopper, Grace Murray," p. 356.

## REFERENCES

Williams, Kathleen Broome. *Grace Hopper: Admiral of the Cyber Sea*. Annapolis, MD: Naval Institute Press, 2004.

Williams, Kathleen Broome. "Hopper, Grace Murray." In *New Dictionary of Scientific Biography*, vol. 3. Detroit: Charles Scribner's Sons/Thomson Gale, 2008, pp. 356–361.

ITEMS EXHIBITED

113. "Lt. Hopper at desk in the Computation Lab." Photograph. Cambridge, MA, Harvard University, 1947. (Courtesy, Grace Murray Hopper Collection, Archives Center, National Museum of American History, Smithsonian Institution.) [SEE FIG. 23]

114. The Staff of the Computation Laboratory. *A Manual of Operation for the Automatic Sequence Controlled Calculator*. Cambridge: Harvard University Press, 1946.

This manual for the first large-scale automatic calculator, put into operation in 1944 at Harvard, is generally regarded as the first publication on digital computing. Grace Murray Hopper, a U.S. Navy lieutenant with a Ph.D. in mathematics, was the principal author. Throughout the 561-page volume are the earliest examples of sequences of arithmetic operations for numerical problems. The *Manual* was the first of a series of more than thirty publications on computer technology by Harvard during this early period in the development of digital computing.

115. Howard H. Aiken and Grace M. Hopper. "The Automatic Sequence Controlled Calculator." Parts I, II and III. *Electrical Engineering*, vol. 65, nos. 8-9, 10, and 11, pp. 384–391, 449–454, and 522–528 (August-September, October, and November 1946). Issues in wrappers.

The three issues of this serial contain a condensed version of the Harvard publication *A Manual of Operation for the Automatic Sequence Controlled Calculator*. Although Hopper was the chief programmer of the machine and wrote much of the book, the name of her supervisor, the person who initiated the computing project at Harvard, appears as the first author. The article is the first published description of the Mark I to reach a wide audience.

116. Grace Murray Hopper. "The Education of a Computer." In *Proceedings of the 1952 Association for Computing Machinery Meeting*, Pittsburgh, May 2–3, 1952, pp. 243–249. Pittsburgh: Richard Rimbach Associates, 1952. (Courtesy, P. J. Mode.)

Grace Hopper's most important contributions to computing were programming concepts. In this paper, she predicted, correctly, that programming, not hardware, would be the future limitation in digital computing. She addressed this problem by creating a program that used the computer itself to translate, i.e., "compile," instructions written in a non-specialist's language to instructions that the computer could implement. In this milestone article, she explains this idea and many other innovative concepts that soon came to fruition.

# THE MEDICAL SCIENCES

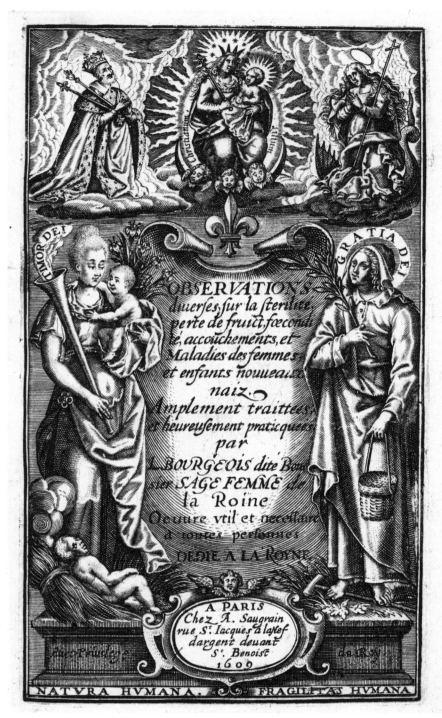

Fig. 24. Title page of Louise Bourgeois Boursier. *Observations Diverses, sur la Sterilité, perte de Fruict, Foecondité, Accouchements, et Maladies des Femmes, et Enfants Nouveaux Naiz.* Paris: Chez A. Saugrain, 1609. (Courtesy, Cushing/Whitney Medical Library, Yale University.) [CAT. 118]

# LOUISE BOURGEOIS BOURSIER  1563–1636

## BIOGRAPHY

Born in a Parisian suburb, Louise Bourgeois had a girl's limited education in reading, writing, and needlepoint, nothing to point her toward her remarkable career in the practice and teaching of obstetrics and gynecology. Her marriage in 1584 to Martin Boursier, a military barber surgeon who worked with Ambroise Paré, First Surgeon to the King, whose reputation rested in part on his use of his own observations, brought her close to medicine and to the highest intellectual and influential levels of her society.

During the siege of Paris by Henry IV in 1589, with her husband away on military duty and needing a living for herself and her three children, she supplemented her paltry needlework income by serving as a midwife in her Left Bank neighborhood, and in 1598, passing a rigorous license examination by a physician, two surgeons, and two midwives, became an official midwife.

Through her skill, assertiveness and good fortune, she became the midwife for several prominent noblewomen and finally of Queen Marie de Medici. Boursier delivered five children for the queen, her first in 1601, the boy who became Louis XIII, at whose birth she correctly identified the cause of suckling difficulty which was then cured surgically.[1] The king as well as the queen appreciated her and compensated her well: eventually the king, speaking to her with friendly warmth, awarded her in addition to the substantial moneys she had earned, a yearly pension of 300 écus, far above an average midwife's earnings, with 500 écus for birthing any of their future male children and 300 écus for any future females. This was in addition, he reminded her, to whatever she earned from other noble births, and from the 200 écus the queen herself gifted her on occasion.

In her great work, *Observations Diverses sur la Sterilité, perte de Fruict, Foecondité, Accouchements, et Maladies des Femmes, et Enfants Nouveaux Naiz*, first published in 1609, she wrote with pride that she was the first woman practicing her art to take up the pen. Her book was immediately translated into the major European languages, published in several subsequent editions, and became the essential reference for over a century.

Her vastly inclusive content touches all contingencies as she had herself experienced them. She presents instruction and guidelines for both normal and high-risk deliveries; describes how in cases with severe hemorrhage or certain other situations birth can be enabled by podalic version, that is by turning the fetus so that one or both feet present through the cervix; how to deliver a child from a mother who is dying; how to deliver twins when the mother is exhausted, and many other dire and life-threatening situations. She negates the myth that twins of the same sex do not survive. She discusses ways of handling placental retention, and describes the importance of maintaining a proper and safe environment during labor, particularly pertinent at a time when birthing was a social affair with relatives and neighbors in the delivery room. Her writing covers both prepartum and postpartum care. In her encyclopedic study of obstetrics and perinatal medicine, she produced a compendium that saved thousands of lives of mothers and infants, and stood the test of time.

Then her career met a great crisis. On June 5, 1627, Marie de Bourbon-Montpensier, sister-in-law of now King Louis XIII, died a week after having delivered. The brief autopsy report, though coming to no definite conclusions, describes what appears to be severe peritonitis and also notes a small piece of placenta firmly attached to the left side of the uterus. The implication of this last finding – especially for Boursier's jealous enemies at court – was that the midwife's care had caused the death. She defended herself vigorously in a twenty-three-page book.[2] Noting the autopsy's flaws, she points out that if a piece of placenta had been retained, it would have been washed out with the excessive bleeding which commonly accompanies partial placental retention. The autopsy places the placental fragment *opposite* the location of the infection and distended, necrotic bowel. Further, she notes, those signing the autopsy report lacked experience with obstetrics and/or, as the very physicians who cared for Marie de Bourbon during her pregnancy, had reason to shift the blame toward the delivery. It was well attested that the patient had been seriously ill during the pregnancy, having required several bloodlettings. The response to her book, attributed to the Royal Surgeon,[3] evading Boursier's strong argument about the retained placenta, attacks her by saying that the peritonitis could have been caused by several actions the midwife may have carried out including rough treatment during delivery, binding the abdomen too tight, too much pressure on the uterus to extract the placenta, etc.

Current consideration of the scant and dubious autopsy report indicates that the attached placental fragment, had it not washed out with blood, could only have been removed by surgical procedures then unavailable. Most pertinent for Boursier, since infection isn't mentioned near the retained piece of placenta, the mortality is ascribable to peritonitis secondary to bowel necrosis on the opposite side. In terms of malpractice, the defendant is not guilty. Following this episode, however, Boursier left the court, continuing her practice and working on several books until her death in 1636.

Like the best physicians, she never stopped learning: "There has never been complete mastery in medicine, nor in all that depends on it; one must learn until the last day of one's life . . . "[4]

## SIGNIFICANT CONTRIBUTIONS

Boursier's observations of her thousands of cases, and rejection of rote dependence on past practices, led her to discover, publish and disseminate evidence-based obstetrics, written in the vernacular. Her works, based upon rational understanding of care during pregnancy, delivery and post partum, resulted in saving countless lives and averted many family tragedies.

She played a significant role in the long and continuing process of women's liberation by lifting from women a burden they carried from the Bible: the admonition to Eve that she will bear children in pain. It was thought that pain occurs to women in labor as atonement for Eve's sin. Empiricist that she was, woman that she was, and a true healer, Louise Boursier denied that that there was any value – any paying for sin – in the pains of childbirth. Thus she was a giant in helping to alleviate physical pain, fear and mortality, and the burdens of low self-esteem and guilt.

RJR AND YK

## ENDNOTES

1. Robert J. Ruben. "Development of Otorhinological Care of the Child." *Acta Otolaryngologica*, vol. 124, no. 4 (2004), pp. 536–539.

2. See Louise Bourgeois Boursier, 1627 (cat. no. 122).

3. Charles Guillemeau (attributed). *Remonstrame à Madame Bourcier, touchant son Apologie, contre le Rapport que les Medecins ont fait, de ce qui a causé la Mort déplorable de MADAME.* Paris: J. Jacquin, 1627.

4. Translated from Louise Bourgeois Boursier, *Observations* part III, 1626, pp. 37–38.

## REFERENCES

Hurd-Mead, Kate Campbell. *A History of Women in Medicine. From the Earliest Times to the Beginning of the Nineteenth Century.* Haddam, CT: Haddam Press, 1938.

Long, Kathleen P. *Gender and Scientific Discourse in Early Modern Culture.* Farnham, Surrey: Ashgate Publishing, 2010.

Perkins, Wendy. *Midwifery and Medicine in Early Modern France: Louise Bourgeois.* Exeter: University of Exeter Press, 1996.

117. Louise Bourgeois Boursier (1563–1636), royal midwife. Engraving from Boursier, *Observations Diverses, sur la Sterilité, Perte de Fruict, Foecondité, Accouchements, et Maladies des Femmes, et Enfants Nouveaux Naiz*. Paris: A. Saugrain, 1609. (Courtesy, The Cushing/Whitney Medical Library, Yale University.)

118. Louise Bourgeois Boursier. *Observations Diverses, sur la Sterilité, Perte de Fruict, Foecondité, Accouchements, et Maladies des Femmes, et Enfants Nouveaux Naiz*. Paris: Chez A. Saugrain, 1609. (Courtesy, Cushing/Whitney Medical Library, Yale University.)
[SEE FIG. 24]

In this first edition of the first published book on obstetrics by a woman, Boursier relies on observations of over 2000 deliveries, abandoning untested dogma. Writing in the vernacular, not Latin, enabled the dissemination of her ideas. It was thought at the time that women's pain in labor is atonement for Eve's sin. Boursier denied that that there was any paying for sin in the pains of childbirth. She was a giant in helping to alleviate the pain, fear and mortality of childbirth, and the burden of low self-esteem and guilt.

119. Louise Bourgeois Boursier. *Observations Diverses, sur la Sterilité, Perte de Fruict, Foecondité, Accouchements, et Maladies des Femmes, et Enfants Nouveaux Naiz*. Paris: Chez A. Saugrain, 1617. (Courtesy, The National Library of Medicine.)

This second edition of Boursier's widely read book on obstetrics includes a powerful new section entitled "Instruction à ma fille" [Advice to my daughter]. Here the midwife addresses her own unborn daughter, and beyond that, all midwives – *all* her daughters – describing their ethical responsibilities to the women under their care. A token of her broadmindedness and purposeful focus on the health of her patients is her advice that the midwife should not hide good remedies from physicians. They should share freely and explain rationally their knowledge.

120. Louise Bourgeois Boursier. *Observations Diverses, sur la Sterilité, Perte de Fruict, Foecondité, Accouchements, et Maladies des Femmes, et Enfants Nouveaux Naiz*. Rouen: Thomas Daré, 1626. (Courtesy, The New York Academy of Medicine Library.)

In 1626, Boursier expanded her book on obstetrics, published by Thomas Daré in Paris as the third edition, and again in Rouen in this, the fourth edition. She provides greater detail in her descriptions and treatments of gynecological and obstetrical issues and problems. She includes a step-by-step guideline for care from prenatal through delivery and ends with postnatal regimes. She details the management of both the normal and abnormal course of a pregnancy. Open to title page with engraving of King Henry

IV and Queen Marie de Medici kneeling on either side of the enthroned Madonna and Christ Child.

121. Louise Bourgeois Boursier. *Recit Veritable de la Naissance de Messeigneurs et Dames les Enfans de France: avec les Particularitez qui y ont esté, et Pouvoient estre Remarquées.* Paris: Chez Melchior Mondiere, 1626. (Courtesy, The New York Academy of Medicine Library.)

In describing with immediacy the details of noble births she attended, Boursier reveals her on the spot responses to birthing travails. A remarkable picture emerges of the trust and love she enjoyed from Marie de Medici and King Henry IV who, at a frustrating moment, put his hand on her shoulder. Open to pages 160–161: at the end of a long, painful episode, to which the King was closely attentive, "he raised his eyes to heaven with his hands in prayer and gave thanks to God. The tears ran down his face, big as large weights."

122. Louise Bourgeois Boursier. *Apologie de Louyse Bourgeois dite Bourcier, sage Femme de la Royne Mere du Roy, & de seu Madame. Contre le Rapport des Medecins.* Paris: Chez Melchior Mondiere, 1627. (Courtesy, The New York Academy of Medicine Library.)

When a member of the royal family died after delivery with Boursier in attendance, her jealous enemies at court were quick to blame her. She wrote this book in her own defense, noting the flawed autopsy report concocted to dishonor her. The response to her book, probably written by the Royal Surgeon, is an unconvincing array of unproved allegations. The evidence vindicates Boursier but she left court following this episode. Open to title page.

123. Louise Bourgeois Boursier. *The Compleat Midwife's Practice Enlarged.* London: Printed for Nath. Brook at the Angel in Corn-hill, 1663. (Courtesy, The National Library of Medicine.)

Boursier's book, a fundamental source for obstetrics into the eighteenth century, was translated into many languages including Latin – an irony given that her original vernacular increased the availability of her ideas. This third English edition includes a guide for conceiving, bearing and nursing children derived from the experience of English practitioners. Open to Plate 1: the illustration, with its respect for feminine modesty – twigs and branches in the "right places" – pictures a "natural," that is a normal position of the fetus in the womb.

# MARY CORINNA PUTNAM JACOBI  1842–1906

## BIOGRAPHY

Mary Corinna Putnam was born August 31, 1842 in London, the child of Victorine Putnam and George Putnam, partner of Wiley and Putnam publishing house, who was in London recruiting authors. On her father's side she was a descendant of the seventeenth-century Putnams from Salem, Massachusetts and on her mother's side, a Mayflower descendant. With the family's return to New York in 1847, Putnam established his own publishing company, G. P. Putnam.

Mary was home schooled, as was common at the time, and intellectually enriched through meeting many of her father's literary colleagues. A friend's letter gives a glimpse of her at age eight as the precocious author of "Robinson Crusoe's Farmyard."[1] At fifteen she entered the newly established public and progressive Twelfth Street School in Manhattan that fostered confidence and independence for girls. In 1860, at age seventeen, she published her first of eight published stories, "Found and Lost," for which she received $18.[2]

That year she began her medical career by attending clinics of Elizabeth Blackwell, the first American female physician, whose example inspired Mary for the rest of her life. Finding the doors to the established medical schools in the United States closed to women, however, she matriculated into the New York College of Pharmacy (turning down her father's offer to pay her $250, the pharmacy school tuition, if she would stay at home), becoming its first woman graduate in 1863, in the midst of the Civil War. Her thesis was "Dialysis."

In that same year she formally resigned from the church, unable to reconcile rationality with belief, and traveled to New Orleans to care for her brother, a Union officer who had contracted malaria;[3,4] here she witnessed the horrors of war and the desperate plight of the freedmen. Upon returning north, she matriculated at the Female Medical College of Pennsylvania but, dissatisfied with what she recognized as an inferior education, went to Paris seeking a scientifically based medical education. There, however, the École de Médecine, in 1866, turned her down, the reason recorded: for a woman to practice medicine in France "seems so contrary to our customs and social conditions."[5] She persisted, though, and eventually became the first woman permitted to attend class at the École de Médecine, although non-matriculating and with the requirement that she enter the classroom by a separate door and sit alone near the professor. In 1868, the school relented, allowing her to matriculate, and she became the first woman accepted by the École. Living through the siege of Paris, she graduated in July 1871, receiving a bronze medal for her thesis, *De la Graisse neuter et des Acides gras* (Of Neutral Fat and Fatty Acids).[6]

Upon her return to New York in 1871, she obtained a position at the Women's Medical College of the New York Infirmary, caring for patients, teaching, and carrying out research. In the same year, she became a member of the New York Academy of Medicine through the liberalness of its president, Abraham Jacobi, a leader in American pediatrics and a founder of the American Communist Party. Mary Putnam married Abraham Jacobi in 1873, continuing her medical research, teaching, and clinical work, while becoming a powerful advocate for the rights of women and children. She died of a brain tumor in 1906. Sir William Osler in his eulogy said:

> The scientific character of her numerous contributions gave a new distinction to the work of women physicians in this country, and contributed not a little to allay the strong animus which for so long kept them out of schools and medical societies. That almost everywhere the door is now open is due largely to her influence exerted unconsciously in this way.[7]

## SIGNIFICANT CONTRIBUTIONS

For Mary Putnam Jacobi, correlations did not prove causation, a radical concept at the time (and one still capable of causing misleading confusion in medicine). By example and teaching, she brought the scientific method to American medicine. She based her work on experimentally provable, objective, observable and repeatable physiological observations. The outcome of her scientific approach is conveyed in her studies of female physiology, published in her book, *The Question of Rest for Women during Menstruation*.[8] Here she demonstrated that, contrary to the "com-

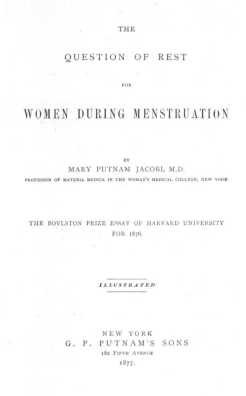

Fig. 25. Title page of Mary Putnam Jacobi, M.D., *The Question of Rest for Women during Menstruation,* New York: G. P. Putnam's Sons, 1877, of the published manuscript for which she received Harvard University's Boylston Prize in 1876. [CAT. 127]

mon sense" assumptions of the time, menstruation did not impede nor diminish the abilities of women to carry on intellectual actives. For this work, she received in 1876 one of the highest awards in medicine of the time, the Boylston Prize from Harvard.[9] Her work is the foundation upon which rests the inclusion of women in higher education and the professions.

Among the earliest medical researchers to focus on the area of pediatric neurology, her article "Pathology of Infantile Paralysis" identifies the location of the underlying lesion in a motor neuron,[10] a discovery that led to the development of the polio vaccine seventy-five years later. In her prescient book, *Physiological Notes on Primary Education and the Study of Language*, based upon her understanding derived through experiment and observation, she vastly enlarged understanding of the essential question of how children learn – leading to significant insights into how children *best* learn. In many ways, education today is still catching up with Mary Putnam Jacobi.[11]

RJR AND YK

## ENDNOTES

1. George Haven Putnam. *A Memoir of George Palmer Putnam: Together with a Record of the Publishing House founded by Him*. New York and London: G. P. Putnam and Sons, 1903, p. 256.

2. Mary C. Putnam, "Found and Lost" (cat. no. 125).

3. Bittel, p. 32.

4. *Life and Letters*, p. 58.

5. Bittel, p. 63.

6. Mary C. Putnam, *Thèse pour Le Doctorat en Médecine* (cat. no. 126).

7. *In Memory of Mary Putnam Jacobi*, p. 3 (cat. no. 130).

8. Mary Putnam Jacobi, 1877 (cat. no. 127).

9. Harvard Medical School first admitted women in 1945.

10. Mary Putnam Jacobi. "Pathology of Infantile Paralysis." *The American Journal of Obstetrics and Diseases of Women and Children*, vol. 7 (1874), pp. 1–44.

11. Mary Putnam Jacobi, 1899 (cat. no. 129).

## REFERENCES

Bittel, Carla. *Mary Putnam Jacobi and the Politics of Medicine in Nineteenth-Century America*. Chapel Hill: The University of North Carolina Press, 2009.

Jacobi, Mary P. *Stories and Sketches*. New York and London: G. P. Putnam's Sons, Knickerbocker Press, 1907.

Putnam-Jacobi, Mary P. *"Common Sense" Applied to Woman Suffrage*. New York: G. P. Putnam's Sons, 1894.

Putnam, Ruth, ed. *Life and Letters of Mary Putnam Jacobi*. New York and London: G. P. Putnam's Sons, The Knickerbocker Press, 1925.

Truax, Rhoda. *The Doctors Jacobi*. Boston: Little, Brown and Company, 1952.

## ITEMS EXHIBITED

124. Mary Putnam Jacobi, pioneer in women's health and pediatric neurology. Photograph ca. 1866. (Courtesy, Prints and Photographs Division, The Library of Congress.)

125. Mary C. Putnam. "Found and Lost," *The Atlantic Monthly,* vol. 30, pp. 391–407 (April 1860). Single issue.

Mary Putnam's first published work, written when she was seventeen, is a moralistic adventure story that takes place in North Africa, replete with ancient Egyptian tombs, kidnappings, storms and dramatic rescues.

126. Mary C. Putnam. *Thèse pour Le Doctorat en Médecine, Présentée et soutenue le 23 Juillet 1871, Par Mary – C. Putnam née Londres. De la graisse neutre et des acides gras. 1871.* Paris: A. Parent, Imprimeur de la Faculté de Médecine, 31 Rue, Monsieur-le-Prince, 24, 1871. (Courtesy, Health Sciences Library, University of North Carolina at Chapel Hill.)

Mary Putnam's doctoral thesis, "On neutral fat and fatty acids," was one requirement for her medical degree at the École de Médecine in Paris. In this thesis, she applies chemistry and physiology in addition to pathology for the understanding of disease processes. It is interesting that in spite of the difficulties the institution placed in her way to attend, and then to matriculate, it saw its way to acknowledging the excellence of this thesis by awarding it a bronze medal.

127. Mary Putnam Jacobi, M.D. *The Question of Rest for Women during Menstruation.* New York: G. P. Putnam's Sons, 1877. [SEE FIG. 25]

Jacobi reversed the assumption that menstruation diminished a woman's intellectual abilities, arguing from objective measures of pulse rate, blood pressure and temperature. "There is nothing in the nature of menstruation to imply necessity, or even the desirability, of rest for women whose nutrition is really normal." The manuscript, submitted under a pseudonym so as not to be discounted because it was written by a woman, received Harvard University's Boylston Prize in 1876, which led to the book's publication. Open to pages 156–157: the illustrations demonstrate Jacobi's quantitative approach, here applied to tracing pulse pressure in the course of menstruation.

128. Mary Putnam Jacobi. Autograph letter to Toni and Sophie Boas, February 27, 1884. (Courtesy, The New York Academy of Medicine Library.)

Both of Jacobi's children, Marjorie and Ernst, contracted diphtheria in the summer of 1883. Marjorie survived but Ernst died in June at age seven. Still grieving eight months later, and concerned for her husband, she writes to her friends Toni and Sophie Boas, "It seemed very hard to go on doing the same things after Ernst was gone – the loss of this darling boy has been so overwhelmingly terrible to the doctor, that I have scarcely dared to think of myself."

129. Mary Putnam Jacobi, M.D. *Physiological notes on primary education and the study of language*. New York: Putnam, 1899.

In this work, Jacobi pioneers the application of science, including statistics, psychology and neurology, toward optimizing primary school education and the effective acquisition of language skills. Based upon her understanding derived through experiment and observation, she vastly enlarged understanding of how children learn – leading to significant insights into how children best learn. Open to pages 68 and 69: the illustration demonstrates the areas of the brain that were known at the time to mediate speech, language and hearing.

130. *In Memory of Mary Putnam Jacobi. Memorial at New York Academy of Medicine, January 4, 1907*. New York: New York Academy of Medicine, Knickerbocker Press, 1907.

The collected tributes to Mary Putnam Jacobi by speakers at her memorial service at the New York Academy of Medicine. Contributors include Dr. William Osler, Regius Chair of Medicine at Oxford, Dr. Felix Adler, professor of political and social ethics at Columbia, social reformer and a founder of the Society for Ethical Culture, Florence Kelley, a political reformer who worked against sweatshops and for the minimum wage, eight-hour work-days, and children's rights, and Dr. Emily Blackwell a leader in establishing the rights of women to become physicians. Open to page 3, Dr. Osler's Introduction.

# HELEN BROOKE TAUSSIG  1898–1986

## BIOGRAPHY

To arrive at her great achievements, Helen Taussig had much to overcome – the early death of her mother, dyslexia, severe hearing impairment and the discrimination of much of the medial establishment – but she had a strong suit: she came from a family with a distinguished academic father, and her mother was highly educated as well.

Taussig was born in Cambridge, Massachusetts in 1898 to Frank W. Taussig, an eminent Harvard professor of economics, and Edith Thomas Guild, daughter of an established New England family who had graduated from the "Radcliffe Annex," but who died when Helen was eleven years old. Overcoming severe dyslexia, Helen matriculated as one of the first students in what is now Radcliffe College, but seeking broader social and educational experience, she transferred to the University of California, Berkeley and graduated in 1921.

Determined to study medicine, she was forced, like so many others, to travel the long way round to fulfill her goal, and to swallow some pride on the journey. Since Harvard Medical School would not accept a woman (first doing so only in 1945) she applied to Harvard School of Public Health, which allowed her to attend classes but would not award her a degree. She was also allowed to study histology at the Harvard Medical School but with a caveat: she was kept in a room by herself so as "to not contaminate" the male students.

She finally found a sympathetic mentor in Alexander Begg, professor of anatomy at Boston University, who led her to study isolated heart muscle contractions. This resulted in her first publication and set the stage for her life's work in cardiology.[1] Even with her major publication, Harvard Medical School would not permit her to matriculate, so she applied to The Johns Hopkins School of Medicine, admitted as a function of the legacy of Mary Elizabeth Garrett and the Women's Fund Committee that stipulated that women be accepted on the same terms as men, and she graduated from Hopkins in 1927.

As a pediatric cardiologist, she carefully observed her patients, listened to their hearts, studied their x-rays and fluoroscopies and, when they died, examined their hearts at autopsy. Her precise records and correlation of observations made possible accurate diagnosis and understanding of pathological cardiac physiology resulting from congenital malformations. Her studies led her to design an operation to solve a problem of post-birth anoxia, the Blalock-Taussig procedure, known as "the blue baby operation," that has saved countless infants from death.

It is striking that this outstanding pediatric cardiologist of the twentieth century could not hear the heart sounds of her patients because she suffered from a progressive hearing loss; she compensated by feeling the vibrations of the heart in the child's chest (by the late 1950s she had a portable amplified stethoscope). In recognition of her 1947 landmark book, *Congenital Malformations of the Heart*,[2] she received in 1954 the Albert Lasker Award for outstanding contribution to medicine. In 1959, she was appointed to the position she aspired to, becoming Hopkins' first woman full professor in clinical medicine. She was awarded the Presidential Medal of Freedom by President Lyndon Johnson in 1964, and was elected the first female president of the American Heart Association in 1965. Formal retirement did not end her research: she had just begun a study of defects in the hearts of birds at the time of her death from a car accident in 1986.

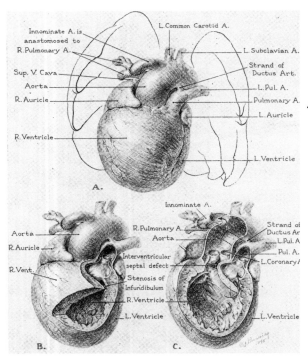

Fig. 26. Helen Brooke Taussig. *Congenital Malformations of the Heart*. New York: The Commonwealth Fund, 1947, showing Fig. 39, the tetralogy of Fallot. Her analysis of this congenital heart malformation led Helen Taussig to design the Blalock-Taussig "blue baby" operation. [CAT. 136]

## SIGNIFICANT CONTRIBUTIONS

If Helen Taussig were a man, we would call her the father of pediatric cardiology – how interesting that to call her "the mother of pediatric cardiology" doesn't have the same ring to it. Her landmark book, *Congenital Malformations of the Heart*, and in its second 1960 edition, is the foundation for pediatric cardiology worldwide, and remains the most comprehensive book on the subject.

Taussig's observation and reasoning led her to design surgical procedures to cure or ameliorate congenital cardiac malformations. Many newborns with a cardiac malformation called the "tetralogy of Fallot" show no signs and symptoms of anoxia – blue lips and rapid exhaustion – until several months after birth. From this, she inferred that the anoxia was caused by the blood not reaching the lungs in sufficient quantity, and so the children died from a lack of oxygen, not from heart failure. For many cases, she was also able to link the onset of anoxia with another congenital malformation, a patent ductus arteriosus that allows blood to reach the lungs for a limited period of time. The ductus typically closes at birth but in problematic instances it remains open, continuing to send blood to the lungs, so that as the ductus gradually closes, the infants with the tetralogy of Fallot become increasingly anoxic. She surmised that if blood could be permanently sent to the lungs, bypassing the cardiac malformation, the children would be cured, so she designed a daring and radical operation, creation of a ductus arteriosus. Not herself a surgeon, she offered the idea to Robert Gross in Boston, the first to surgically close the ductus, but he rejected her plan. She then turned to a new professor of surgery at Hopkins, Alfred Blalock, who, with his research partner, Vivien Thomas, experimented with creating an artificial ductus in dogs by attaching the subclavian artery to the pulmonary artery.[3] Thomas worked for two years developing Taussig's procedure, Blalock observing and assisting. The first human patient underwent the Blalock-Taussig "blue baby operation" in November 1944, with additional procedures following; the report was published May 19, 1945 in the *Journal of the American Medical Association*.[4] This procedure was the beginning of cardiac surgery now commonplace.

In the early 1960s, thalidomide was prescribed widely to pregnant woman for "morning sickness" before thalidomide was linked to the rise in cases of the congenital malformation phocomelia, stunting or absence of arms and/or legs. Taussig conferred in Germany with physicians who had correlated the tremendous increase in phocomelia cases with thalidomide's use in pregnancy and brought the information back to the United States, bringing a fast end to the use of thalidomide and preventing untold numbers of these crippling malformations.[5]

RJR AND YK

ENDNOTES

1. Taussig, 1925 (cat. no. 132).

2. Taussig, 1947 (cat. no. 136).

3. Thomas, Vivien. *Partners of the Heart: Vivien Thomas and his Work with Alfred Blalock: An Autobiography*. Philadelphia: University of Pennsylvania Press, 1998.

4. Blalock, 1945 (cat. no. 134).

5. Taussig, 1962 (cat. no. 137).

REFERENCES

Baldwin, Joyce. *To Heal the Heart of a Child: Helen Taussig, M.D.* New York: Walker and Company, 1992.

McCabe, B. Helen Taussig. http://archive.magazine.jhu.edu/2011/08/helen-taussig (accessed 05/29/2012).

ITEMS EXHIBITED

131. Helen Taussig with a pediatric "blue baby" patient in a wheelchair, and child's mother (note that the child's lips are dark from anoxia). Photograph. (Courtesy, Alan Mason Chesney Medical Archives, Johns Hopkins Medical Institutions.)

132. Helen Brooke Taussig and Faith L. Meserve. "Rhythmic Contractions in Isolated Strips of Mammalian Ventricle." *American Journal of Physiology*, vol. 52, pp. 89–98 (1925). Bound volume. (Courtesy, The New York Academy of Medicine.)

   Taussig's first publication, reporting the research done at Boston University before she was a medical student, and appearing in a major journal while she was a medical student, set the course of her life's work in the study of heart function. It is a substantial contribution in basic science for understanding the contractility of cardiac muscle. Open to Figs. 1 through 5 that show spontaneous contractions of heart muscle in several species (Figs. 1 through 3 and 5) and the response of heart muscle to adrenalin (Fig. 4).

133. Taussig's "blue-baby" operation follow-up form with handwritten annotations by a patient's parent, two pages, lender's collection reference 0179205, 1945. Facsimile. (Courtesy, Alan Mason Chesney Medical Archives, Johns Hopkins Medical Institutions.)

   Taussig followed up post-operatively her patients by sending this form to parents on a regular basis, and it informed her of the long-term outcome of the procedure. The results became part of her classic book (cat. no. 136). While it is known that she used the data for scientific purposes, one must pause to suppose that when she read a parent's words about a child such as, "She plays hard, as if trying to make up for lost time," she would have found a well-earned sense of gratification.

134. Alfred Blalock and Helen Brooke Taussig. "The Surgical Treatment of Malformations of the Heart in which there is Pulmonary Stenosis or Pulmonary Atresia." *Journal of the American Medical Association*, vol. 128, pp. 189–202 (May 19, 1945). Offprint.

   Taussig's studies led her to design an operation to solve a fatal problem of post-birth anoxia, the Blalock-Taussig procedure that became widely known as "the blue baby operation." This is the first cardiac operation to reconstruct a congenital malformation ever developed, and one that since first performed on November 29, 1944, has saved countless infants from early death. This is the initial report of the first three successful cases. Open to Fig. 1, a diagram of the operation.

135. Helen Brooke Taussig. X-ray, and drawings of heart and blood flow paths used to illustrate *Congenital Malformations of the Heart* (cat. no. 136), lender's collection reference 0179065. (Courtesy, Alan Mason Chesney Medical Archives, Johns Hopkins Medical Institutions.)

Taussig designed this sheet, showing the layout of a plate describing a congenitally malformed heart, for her book *Congenital Malformations of the Heart* (cat. no. 136). Taussig combined four representations of the same heart, an x-ray (UL), a drawing of the external appearance (UR), the heart opened showing single ventricle and insufficient outlet chamber (LL), and the course of circulation (LR). The visual material appears in the published book but not on a single plate.

136. Helen Brooke Taussig. *Congenital Malformations of the Heart*. New York: The Commonwealth Fund, 1947. [SEE FIG. 26]

This is the first edition of Taussig's landmark book on pediatric cardiology, which resulted in the diagnosis and cure of innumerable congenital malformations. This book had an immediate and vast influence on pediatric cardiology worldwide, and led to her receiving the Lasker Award, medicine's highest award. Open to pages 223–224 that illustrate, on p. 223, two x-rays with different views of the same infant's heart and, on p. 224, her brilliant analyses of the x-rays as transmitted through her own line drawings.

137. Helen Brooke Taussig. "A Study of the German outbreak of Phocomelia. The Thalidomide Syndrome." *Journal of the American Medical Association*, vol. 180, pp. 1106–1114 (June 30, 1962). Offprint.

In the early 1960s, the sedative thalidomide was prescribed widely to pregnant woman to allay "morning sickness." Taussig brought to the United States German data that identified thalidomide as the cause of phocomelia – congenital stunting or absence of arms and legs – leading to the ban on the use of thalidomide in the United States, and preventing untold number of these crippling malformations. Open to pages 1106 and 1107 showing the epidemiology (Table 1) and the severe congenital malformation caused by the drug (Figs. 1–2).

# FLORENCE RENA SABIN   1871–1953

BIOGRAPHY

"Of course I'll stay. I have research in progress," Florence Sabin said when Johns Hopkins School of Medicine passed her over for a man less distinguished as chairman of the Department of Anatomy. *Research in progress*: that's where Sabin's heart and head were. That was the priority that drove her monumental discoveries in how the body fights pathogens that, today, form the foundation of our understanding of immunity.

Sabin was born November 9, 1871 in Central City, Colorado, to George Sabin, a mining engineer whose Huguenot family had emigrated in the seventeenth century and Serena Sabin, a Confederate school teacher who moved to Colorado during the Civil War. Her mother died when Florence was seven, and she and her sister went to live with relatives in Vermont. Graduating from Vermont Academy in Saxtons River, she earned her Bachelor of Science degree in 1893 from Smith College, founded by Sophia Smith " . . . to furnish for my own sex means and facilities for education equal to those which are afforded now in our colleges to young men."[1]

In 1892, Mary Garrett's Women's Fund Committee of Baltimore offered $500,000 to enable the opening of Johns Hopkins Medical School with *one condition*: women must be allowed to matriculate; thus, Hopkins became the first co-educational graduate medical school in the United States. Admitted in 1896 and graduating in 1900, Sabin, having already published major work on the medulla and midbrain, was awarded the prestigious and competitive internship at Johns Hopkins Hospital under the famous physician Sir William Osler.

It wasn't what she really wanted. Her passion was research.

Hopkins' medical school, however, would not hire a woman as faculty. Mary Garrett's fund came through with a research fellowship and an $800 stipend for Sabin in the Anatomy Department, where she found a sympathetic mentor in the chairman, Franklin Mall. Appointed assistant in anatomy in 1902, she became the first woman faculty member in the School of Medicine.

Throwing herself into neuroanatomy research, she published in 1901 *An Atlas of the Medulla and Midbrain*, still used today. She then embarked on investigating the vascular system's development, defining the embryology of the lymphatic vessels and establishing the development of many cells found in blood. In 1917, Sabin was

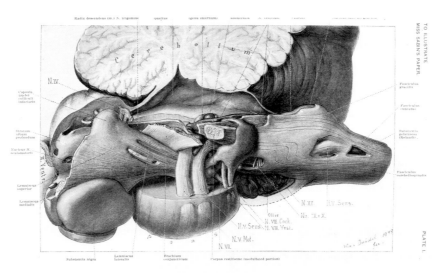

Fig. 27. Florence Rena Sabin. "A Model of the Medulla Oblongata, Pons, and Midbrain of a Newborn Babe." In *Contributions to the Science of Medicine Dedicated by his Pupils to William Henry Welch on the 25th Anniversary of his Doctorate*, pp. 925–1045. Baltimore: Johns Hopkins University Press, 1900. Plate I. [CAT. 140]

appointed professor of histology, the first woman full professor in Johns Hopkins Medical School.

Students remembered her engagement with developing researchers and humorous nature:

> Students who showed an interest in extramural or non medical problems were promptly invited to dine . . . she showed a phenomenal flair for social entertainment in her home, a love for and skill at the art of cookery, and a knack for the preparation of dinners . . . carried on at times with fun and a pleasant burlesque of the exactness of scientific techniques . . . stop watch turning steaks exactly every third minute, on the dot of the 180th second; of scalding the dishes afterwards and cleaning them as though they were to be used for the next experiment in the laboratory.[2]

In 1924 Sabin was elected first woman president of the American Association of Anatomists, and in 1925 became the first woman elected to the National Academy of Sciences.

Johns Hopkins Medical School, however, had not changed much in its resistance to women's professional advancement. In 1919, Sabin, a full professor, was passed over for chairman of the Anatomy Department in favor of an associate professor.[3,4] Her outraged students petitioned for reconsideration and Mary Garrett's Women's Fund Committee complained vigorously. It was at this critical juncture that Sabin, asked if she would stay at the Hopkins following such unfair treatment, replied that she would let nothing stand in the way of her research in progress.

Still, given the terrible slight, there's satisfaction that in 1925 the Rockefeller Institute in New York recruited her as their first full-time faculty member to establish and head the Department of Cellular Studies. Using techniques she had developed in vital staining, she and her group revealed the role of monocytes and other white blood cells in defending the body against pathogens.

Sabin was prescient in organizing an early multi-disciplinary, inter-institutional research effort, integrating bacteriological, chemical, and biological research on tuberculosis carried out in private and governmental institutes, a creative strategy not always reached today.

On April 15, 1936, the young medical researcher Helen Taussig wrote to Sabin, asking whether she, Taussig, should she stay at Hopkins, concerned that the attitude to women faculty would prevent her promotion, and dismayed that she earned less than her male peers. The money wasn't the essential issue, Taussig wrote, " . . . but my self-respect demands that the institution I work in, should have confidence in me." Sabin replied, ". . . my advice to you is to stay where you are and keep on with the work without a troubled mind."[5]

Retiring from the Rockefeller in 1938 and moving back to Colorado, Sabin went on to a game-changing career in public health, her leadership resulting in fundamental legislation, "Sabin Health Laws" for Colorado, which served as a model for other states. She became chairman of the new State Board of Health and the Interim Board of Health and Hospitals of Denver, and manager of the Denver Department of Health and Welfare. In 1952, she was awarded the Albert Lasker Public Service Award for outstanding accomplishments in public health administration.[6]

SIGNIFICANT CONTRIBUTIONS

Sabin demonstrated the anatomy of medulla and midbrain in descriptions that remain the standard. Through her studies of embryology, she demonstrated the origin of the lymphatic system in embryonic veins. Expanding her study of the development of the haemoptoic system by using the new technique of hanging drop tissue culture combined with staining of living tissue (supravital staining), she documented the embryological origin of the many cells that comprise the blood.

This work led to her discovery of a type of cell, the monocyte, and its role in mediating tissue reactions against infection, including tuberculosis, a groundbreaking discovery leading to her investigations of the immune system's processes when confronted by pathogens. In publications that form our current understanding of the basic processes of cellular immunity, she illuminated the mechanisms by which white blood cells react to and destroy pathogens. Florence Sabin's discoveries are today the bases for our understanding of all immunological processes.

RJR AND YK

## ENDNOTES

1. http://www.smith.edu/about_smithtradition.php (accessed January 4, 2013).

2. McMaster, p. 283.

3. *The Johns Hopkins University Medical Department*, p. 75.

4. Florence Rena Sabin. *Franklin Paine Mall: The Story of a Mind*. Baltimore: Johns Hopkins University Press, 1934.

5. Florence Rena Sabin and Helen Brooke Taussig letters, 1936 (cat. no. 144).

6. http://www.laskerfoundation.org/awards/1951public.htm (accessed June 6, 2012).

## REFERENCES

*The Johns Hopkins University Medical Department: Catalogue and Announcement for 1917–1918 (Corrected to October 31, 1917)*. Baltimore: Johns Hopkins Press, 1918.

McMaster, Philip D. and Michael Heidelberger. "Florence Rena Sabin: 1871–1953, A Biographical Memoir," in *Biographical Memoirs*. Washington, DC: National Academies Press, 1960, pp. 269–319.

## ITEMS EXHIBITED

138. Florence Rena Sabin, anatomist and discoverer of immunological processes, at work at the Rockefeller Institute, New York. Photograph by Bachrach. (Courtesy, The American Philosophical Society.)

139. Florence Rena Sabin. "On the Anatomical Relations of the Nuclei of Reception of the Cochlear and Vestibular Nerves." *The Johns Hopkins Hospital Bulletin*, vol. 8, no. 81, pp. 253–259 (1897). Offprint.

During her second year of medical school, using exquisite histological technique and analysis, Sabin differentiated the tissues of two portions of the VIII cranial nerve, the medulla and midbrain, resulting in this, her first publication. Open to Figs. 2 through 5: Figs. 2 through 4 are drawn perpendicular to the axis of the brain stem and Fig. 5 is drawn parallel to the axis of the brain stem.

140. Florence Rena Sabin. "A Model of the Medulla Oblongata, Pons, and Midbrain of a Newborn Babe." In *Contributions to the Science of Medicine Dedicated by his Pupils to William Henry Welch on the 25th Anniversary of his Doctorate*, pp. 925–1045. Baltimore: Johns Hopkins University Press, 1900. Offprint. [SEE FIG. 27]

This festschrift contribution is the first iteration of what would become the trade edition of Sabin's famous *Atlas* of 1901. Open to Plate I, a view of Sabin's three-dimensional model of the medulla oblongata, pons and midbrain of the child, from the aspect of the lateral surface. The drawing of the model, done in 1899, is by the outstanding medical illustrator, Max Brödel, who founded the Department of Medical Illustration at Johns Hopkins Medical Institutions.

141. Florence R. Sabin. *An Atlas of the Medulla and Midbrain: A Laboratory Manual, illustrated with seven color plates, one black plate and forty-two figures.* Henry McElderry Knower, ed. Baltimore: The Friedenwald Company Publishers, 1901.

Sabin's *Atlas*, based on her festschrift text (cat. no. 140), includes a new author's preface explaining the reasons for creating the three-dimensional model, and discusses changes and additions in this 1901 volume: the *Atlas* now has fuller plate references, rearrangement of the contents for ease of use, pertinent citations and – most important – an index. Commercially published, the *Atlas* became broadly disseminated – and it is still in print. Open to Plate III, showing the dorsal surface of the model, as drawn by Max Brödel.

142. Florence R. Sabin. "Healing of End-to-End Intestinal Anastomoses with Especial Reference to the Regeneration of Blood Vessels." *The Johns Hopkins Hospital Bulletin*, vol. 31, no. 355, pp. 289–300 (1920). Offprint.

In these experiments, Sabin examined the tissue repair process. Her immediate goal was to understand the mechanisms of healing in connection with Dr. William Halstead's famous surgical treatment of intestinal lesions. Her studies reveal the cellular mechanisms of repair – growing back together again – and led to improved techniques for surgical closure for enhanced healing, and are thus an early example of "translational" research. Open to Plate LIV, Figs. 1 through 6, showing stages in the healing process.

143. Florence R. Sabin. "Direct Growth of Veins by Sprouting." *Carnegie Institution of Washington, Contributions to Embryology*, vol. 14, no. 65, pp. 1–10 (December 1922). Formerly owned by Cecil K. Drinker, Dean, Harvard Medical School, with Drinker's ink signature and ink name stamp. Offprint.

In studying vein regeneration in connection with wound healing, Sabin demonstrated that in the embryo, sprouts arise in venous endothelium, which advance outward to produce new veins. As she wrote (p. 8), "If veins can regenerate as veins it means we have a much more rational accounting with which vessels are repaired in wound healing." Open to Plate I. Figs. A, B, and C showing vein sprouting in the chicken embryo. Fig. D shows endothelial degeneration.

144. Florence Rena Sabin and Helen Brooke Taussig, letters: Taussig to Sabin April 15, 1936 (manuscript) and Sabin to Taussig April 16, 1936 (typed, with Sabin's signature). (Courtesy, The American Philosophical Society.)

In 1936, Helen Taussig, then a young researcher, wrote to Sabin, concerned that Johns Hopkins' conservative attitude toward women would prevent her promotion, and dismayed that she was paid less than her peers. It's not the money, Taussig writes, but " . . . my self-respect demands that the institution I work in, should have confidence in me." Sabin replies, ". . . I am quite sure that my advice to you is to stay where you are and keep on with the work without a troubled mind."

# BARBARA McCLINTOCK  1902–1992

## BIOGRAPHY

Barbara McClintock earned her Ph.D. in 1927 but, as a woman, could not obtain a permanent research position until 1942: in between, she redefined the nature of the gene from fixed to movable and changeable in discoveries that led to her receiving the Nobel Prize, and that underlie current understanding of genetics and disease. And it all started with a fundamental question: *Why amid the general regularity of rows of corn kernels, are some varied in color and position?*

Perhaps she asked that question because she, herself, began life as something of a square peg in a round hole. Born in Hartford, Connecticut, her early life appears to have been troubled by a lack of acceptance from her mother, a Mayflower descendant and pianist, poet and painter, who sent her away periodically to live with relatives in rural Massachusetts. She was solitary, and when she did play with others, preferred boys' games, such as baseball.

With her family's move to Brooklyn, she attended Erasmus Hall High School, taking a routine job after graduation because her mother thought college would spoil her chances of marrying, but her physician father, returning from World War I, supported her college aspirations, and she matriculated at the Cornell School of Agriculture.

Her freshman year was a time of social awakening: she played banjo with a jazz group, became a leader among women students, and learned Yiddish. Quickly finding her true vocation, science, she undertook a study of the cytogenetics – the study of chromosomes and their genetic content and expression – of the maize plant. After graduation, she was accepted into graduate school in the Department of Agriculture, where she demonstrated that each maize chromosome could be identified by its histological characteristics, and that she could locate the position of the genes on the chromosome, as Thomas Hunt Morgan had done recently for the fruit fly. Receiving her doctorate in 1927, she became an instructor in Cornell's Botany Department, the Agriculture Department refusing to hire a woman as faculty.[1]

In 1931 she published with Harriet Creighton, "A Correlation of Cytological and Genetical Crossing-Over in Zea Mays," a landmark article that established her as a leader in the field of genetics.[2]

She was fascinated with differences in color and distribution of corn kernels, and other anomalies that Mendelian genetics failed to explain. Analyzing an anomaly a colleague presented, she found a solution in a eureka moment which she wrote

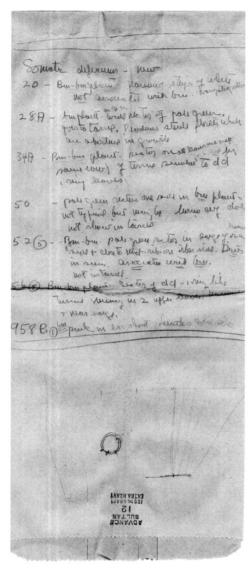

Fig. 28. Barbara McClintock, manuscript on brown paper bag on which she recorded her immediate discovery for the explanation of a significant anomaly as an effect of an extra chromosome, ca. 1929. (Courtesy, The American Philosophical Society.) [CAT. 147]

down on what was at hand – a brown paper bag used to cover corn tassels to control their fertilization.[3] The result was a pair of publications that eventually led to her receiving the Nobel Prize in 1983.[4,5]

Since Cornell's Agriculture Department would not hire a woman for a permanent faculty position, she left, spending five years on fellowships in the United States and Germany; finding the Hitler regime intolerable, she returned to the United States to yet more temporary faculty appointments.

Finally in 1942 she obtained a permanent appointment in the Department of Genetics at the Carnegie Institute of Washington Cold Spring Harbor Laboratories, an ideal position for her since her only responsibility was to carry out research – all she really wanted to do. In 1944 she became the third woman elected to the National Academy of Sciences, received the Lasker Award, and in 1980 was in the first group to receive the MacArthur "genius" Award. She won the Nobel Prize in Physiology in 1983, the first woman awarded the Physiology prize alone, for her discovery of genetic motility.

Although well recognized for her discovery of gene motility, McClintock was more concerned with basic theoretical problems of biology and questions of the genetic processes of control and how these affect the development of individuals and of evolution. As physiologists turned their focus to the molecular biology of phages, viruses and bacteria, she came to feel marginalized for using maize as a cytogenetic model, but new biological tools based on understanding of the molecular structure of DNA and RNA confirmed her cytological observations and calculations and completely vindicated her theories of evolutionary and developmental processes.[6]

Like most great scientists, she was aware of the limits of science. "Oh, yes, you can explain things with physics and chemistry, but you can't explain physics and chemistry. So all you're doing is seeing things in a different light . . . You can get all kinds of relationships . . . You never can find the cause of the cause."[7]

Throughout her career, McClintock was a mentor to many future leaders in genetics. She died shortly after her ninetieth birthday celebration at Cold Spring Harbor, where she was presented with a festschrift with articles by students and colleagues that affirmed much of what she had deduced from cytogenetic studies of corn.[8]

## SIGNIFICANT CONTRIBUTIONS

Barbara McClintock's view of interconnectedness, opening her to new ways of seeing, underlies her revolutionary discoveries. "The point is," she said, "we forget we're all one thing. It's all one. And we're just breaking it up in little things."[9] Her view changed entire concepts of genetics.

Before McClintock's work, genes were considered to be fixed entities like beads on a string; her discovery that genes can move on and around chromosomes was a towering advance. Her further discovery that these translocations are the basis of variation in phenotypes replaced Mendelian genetics, and is the cornerstone of modern genetics. Her discoveries underlie current thinking in the basic biological sciences and in genetic engineering. In the medical realm, her work is the foundation for the development of molecular diagnosis of diseases, the thrust toward personalized medicine, and the search to design individual therapies based upon the modification of genes and their transmission.

From static to dynamic, from fixed to process: this paradigm shift lies at the heart of the modern world, whether one thinks of species or social organizations – or genes. Genes are not fixed, as Mendel thought, but dynamic: Barbara McClintock proved it.

RJR AND YKR

## ENDNOTES

1. McGrayne, p. 152.

2. Harriet B. Creighton and Barbara McClintock. "A Correlation of Cytological and Genetical Crossing-over in Zea Mays." *Proceedings of the National Academy of Sciences USA*, vol. 17 (1931), pp. 492–497.

3. Comfort, p. 55.

4. Barbara McClintock. "The Order of Genes C, Sh, and Wx in Zea Mays with Reference to a Cytologically Known Point in the Chromosome." *Proceedings of the National Academy of Sciences USA*, vol. 17 (1931), pp. 485–491.

5. McClintock, 1948 (cat. no. 148).

6. Comfort, pp. 271–272.

7. Comfort, p. 268.

8. *The Dynamic Genome: Barbara McClintock's Ideas in the Century of Genetics* (cat. no. 151).

9. Comfort, p. 268.

REFERENCES

Comfort, Nathaniel C. *The Tangled Field: Barbara McClintock's Search for the Patterns of Genetic Control.* Cambridge: Harvard University Press, 2001.

Federoff, Nina. "Barbara McClintock: 1902–1992, A Biographical Memoir," in *Biographical Memoirs.* Washington, DC: National Academies Press, 1995, pp. 209–235.

Federoff, Nina and David Botstein, eds. *The Dynamic Genome: Barbara McClintock's Ideas in the Century of Genetics.* Cold Spring Harbor, NY: Cold Spring Harbor Press, 1992.

McGrayne, Sharon Bertsch. *Nobel Prize Women in Science: Their Lives, Struggles and Momentous Discoveries.* New York: Birch Lane Press, 1993, pp. 144–174.

Physiology or Medicine 1983 – Press Release. Nobelprize.org http://nobelprize.org/nobel_prizes/medicine/laureates/1983/press.html (accessed January 24, 2013).

ITEMS EXHIBITED

145. Barbara McClintock, geneticist and 1983 Nobel Laureate. Photograph. (Courtesy, Cold Spring Harbor Laboratory Archives.)

146. Barbara McClintock. "A Cytological and Genetical Study of Triploid Maize." *Genetics*, vol. 14, pp. 180–222 (1929). Offprint. (Courtesy, The American Philosophical Society.)

This article presented the results of McClintock's doctoral dissertation, which became the basis of her life's work. It includes the first published description of a genetic anomaly in a maize plant, the presence of three instead of the usual two chromosomes – a triploid – that McClintock discovered microscopically. Open to pages 184–185. McClintock drew her own illustrations. The discovery is first noted on the brown paper bag (cat. no. 147).

147. Barbara McClintock. Manuscript on brown paper bag, ca. 1929. (Courtesy, The American Philosophical Society.) [SEE FIG. 28]

Scientists placed paper bags over maize flower to prevent uncontrolled fertilization. Working in the field, a colleague was concerned with a pollen's anomalous sterilization rate, but McClintock, excited by the challenge, left immediately for her laboratory to give it thought and shortly returned to the field, shouting, "Eureka." She had figured out that the anomaly was the effect of trisomy, an extra chromosome, and on the spot sketched out her solution on this paper bag. See Fig. 28: "1 ring like trisome running in 2 upper levels" and compare sketch at bottom of the bag.

148. Barbara McClintock. "Mutable Loci in Maize." *Carnegie Institute of Washington Year Book*, vol. 47, pp. 155–169 (1948). Offprint. (Courtesy, Cold Spring Harbor Laboratory Archives.)

This is a key article in McClintock's developing view that the movement of genes creates mutations. Genes moving in and around chromosomes create varying amounts of genetic material at different loci. She observes that variability in the amount of chromosome material determines the intensity of the color of the corn kernel – the greater the number of genetic units, the deeper the color.

149. Ear of Indian maize. (Courtesy, Cold Spring Harbor Laboratory Archives.)

To understand the seemingly random dispersal of the colored kernels, the seeds of maize, and other maize anomalies, McClintock correlated her microscopic histological observations of the plant with the resultant phenotype. This is an example of the maize species McClintock used at Cold Spring Harbor; original maize she examined remains in the Cold Spring Harbor archives.

150. Barbara McClintock. "Chromosome Organization and Genic Expression." *Cold Spring Harbor Symposia and Quantitative Biology*, vol. 16, pp. 13–47 (1951). Offprint. (Courtesy, Cold Spring Harbor Laboratory Archives.)

This breathtaking report shows that mutational changes in appearance arise from the frequent loss of genetic material from a chromosome, and by the presence or absence of other genes. At different times in the course of development, the same chromosome loss causes different effects on the phenotype. Open to pages 22–23, where McClintock explains the observable differences in the corn kernels in Figs. 10 through 15 by a break that occurs in one chromosome, with the differences determined by two variables: the point in developmental time of the break, and the presence or absence of another gene.

151. *The Dynamic Genome: Barbara McClintock's Ideas in the Century of Genetics*. Edited by Nina Fedoroff and David Botstein. Cold Spring Harbor, NY: Cold Spring Harbor Laboratory Press, 1992.

The community of science celebrated McClintock's ninetieth birthday with this festschrift. Each section starts with one of her critical articles and continues with articles by her students and colleagues throughout the world whose work stems from her remarkable observations. Open to her Nobel Prize Lecture of December 8, 1983.

# RITA LEVI-MONTALCINI  1909–2012

## BIOGRAPHY

Rita Levi was born in Turin in 1909 into a prominent Jewish family. Her mother was a painter and her father an electrical engineer who, while encouraging independent thought in his children, believed that women's education should prepare them to serve as mothers and wives.

Nevertheless, Rita sought professional attainment and, stimulated by the death from cancer of a beloved governess, decided to become a doctor. Prevailing upon her father, and with some tutoring, she passed the entrance examinations with the highest scores, and was admitted to the University of Turin medical school, graduating *summa cum laude* in 1936. Taking on her mother's maiden name, Montalcini, so as not to be confused with other high achieving Levis of Turin, she began her specialization in neurology and psychiatry under the guidance of Professor Giuseppe Levi (not of her family).

In 1938, Mussolini's new racial laws prohibited Jews from academic or professional careers, along with other severe strictures. Levi-Montalcini took a position at the Neurological Institute in Brussels but in 1940, just before Germany invaded Belgium, she returned to the relative safety of Turin. There she established her first independent laboratory for the study of embryology using chick models – in the bedroom of the family apartment.

She wanted to reproduce results reported by the embryologist Viktor Hamburger of Washington University in St Louis.[1] Her architect brother built her an incubator and she obtained her experimental material – fertilized chicken eggs – by buying eggs from local farmers to feed her children (though she had none). Her scientific procedure was to surgically remove from the chick embryo (using sewing needles for scalpels) a part, such as a wing, allow the embryo to continue developing in the egg for a determined number of days, then remove the embryo from the egg, and study it histologically with her microscope. What was left of the eggs was used for omelets.

As Turin underwent bombardment, her family fled to a farmhouse in the Piedmont where she reestablished her home laboratory, until 1943, when the Germans occupied northern Italy and the family fled to Florence, taking on an identity as Christians, until the Allied liberation in 1944.

In her studies carried out from 1940 to 1943 she, like Hamburger, observed fewer and smaller neurons in the positions where one would normally find neurons to serve the limb she had excised. Montalcini, however, sampled the specimens over time, while Hamburger had looked at a single end point. Today we would use time-lapse photography, but Levi-Montalcini didn't have time lapse, evading the fascists in her bedroom in the 1940s. Her precise observations of development over time led her to an interpretation completely different from that of Hamburger. Although both observed that excision of a limb resulted in fewer and smaller neurons, Hamburger postulated that the limb somehow stimulated the nerves to grow in their direction, and that without the target limb, the nerves would not migrate there. Levi-Montalcini, in contrast, observed a degenerative process at work: based on her series of specimens obtained at progressive time intervals, she concluded that the neural cells developed, and moved towards the target limb, but that, lacking the target, the cells died, or some became smaller.

Levi-Montalcini published her findings in two publications. The first appeared in 1943, in a Belgian journal, because publication by a Jew was prohibited in Italy, and exquisitely detailed normal development,[2] and the second, in 1944, published in the sovereign Vatican state, showed the degenerative neural effects of removal of the embryonic limb.[3] Viktor Hamburger, now chairman of his department, and eager to explore why the conclusion in her reports differed from his own, invited her for a year at his University: she left Italy in 1947 and remained based in St. Louis for the next three decades.

In 1949, she and Hamburger demonstrated that they had reproduced and validated her observations and conclusions of 1944.[4] That same year Levi-Montalcini demonstrated neural degeneration when an embryonic ear, a sensory organ, was extirpated, rendering her findings now applicable to sensory as well as motor systems.[5]

In 1950 Hamburger brought Levi-Montalcini's attention to a paper by Elmer Bueker, a graduate student, that showed that a mouse tumor, sarcoma 180, when implanted in a chick embryo, caused hypertrophy and hyperplasia of nearby nerve cells.[6] Reproducing and confirming Bueker's observations, Levi-Montalcini hypothesized the presence of a substance which she called a "growth factor," secreted by the tumor, which had two effects: it caused some nerve cells to increase greatly in size, and it caused a dramatic increase in the extrusion of nerve fibers.[7] Through further work in organ culture, she discovered that a substance, secreted by

PLATE II

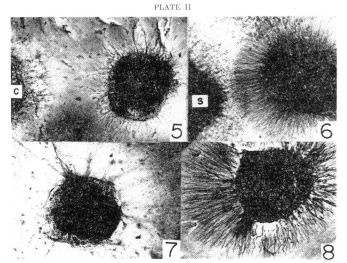

FIGS. 5–8.—Microphotographs of silver-impregnated sensory ganglia, comparing the effect of the intact tumor with the growth-stimulating effect of the cell-free extract of the same time. Fig. 5, control lumbar ganglion of 7-day embryo combined with heart of check embryo (*C*); Fig. 6, ganglion combined with two fragments of sarcoma 37 (*S*); Fig. 7, control ganglion; Fig. 8, ganglion growing in a medium to which the cell-free extract of the tumor was added.

Fig. 29. Figs. 5-8 from Stanley Cohen, Rita Levi-Montalcini, and Viktor Hamburger. "A Nerve Growth-stimulating Factor Isolated from Sarcoma AS 37 and 180." *Proceedings of the National Academy Sciences USA*, vol. 40, no 10, pp. 1014–1018 (1954). Microphotographs of silver-impregnated sensory ganglia, comparing the effect of the intact tumor with the growth stimulating effect of the tumor cell-free extract. Fig. 6 shows nerve cells with stimulated growth in the presence of the tumor. The key is Fig. 8, which shows the nerve growth stimulated with the tumor cell-free extract. Numbers 5 and 7 are controls. [CAT. 156]

the tumor, caused the changes observed in the neural tissue. She also determined that direct contact with the tumor was not necessary, a clue that the substance might work by affecting neighboring cells.

The pressing problem became to define that substance causing the extraordinary neural stimulation. She worked for six years with a biochemist, Stanley Cohen, and in 1954 they succeeded in isolating and purifying the active protein which they called nerve growth factor (NGF)[8]. NGF was the first substance that, through its stimulating properties, could be used to study the growth of nerves. For this work, Rita Levi-Montalcini and Stanley Cohen were jointly awarded the 1986 Nobel Prize in Physiology or Medicine.

Levi-Montalcini studied NGF as a tool for research and in its clinical potential for neurological disorders. She became a full professor at Washington University in 1959, and in 1979 became the director of the Institute of Cell Biology of the Italian National Council of Research in Rome. She received the Albert Lasker Award in 1986, the year of her Nobel Prize. Italy appointed her Senator-for-Life in 2001, where she served until her death at age 103 in 2012.

## SIGNIFICANT CONTRIBUTIONS

Rita Levi-Montalcini's discovery that embryologic nerve cells are physiologically determined to travel to an anatomical unit, and that, target lacking, the cells degenerate, defines our current understanding of neural development. The discovery of nerve growth factor opened new vistas for basic science and medical research. As the Nobel Prize citation recognized:

> Rita Levi-Montalcini and Stanley Cohen have advanced our knowledge from a stage when growth and differentiation could only be described as phenomena and growth factors were unknown, to a situation today when the role of growth factors in cell proliferation, organ differentiation, and tumor transformation is generally recognized.[9]

RJR AND YKR

## ENDNOTES

1. Viktor Hamburger. "The Effects of Wing Bud Extirpation on the Developing Central Nervous System in Chick Embryos." *The Journal of Experimental Zoology*, vol. 63, no. 3 (1934), pp. 449–494.

2. Rita Levi-Montalcini and Giuseppe Levi. "Recherches Quantitatives sur la Marche du Processus de Différenciation des Neurones dans les Ganglions Spinaux de l'Embryon de Poulet." *Archives Biologie Liege*, vol. 54 (1943), pp. 183–206.

3. Rita Levi-Montalcini and Giuseppe Levi. "Correlazioni nello Sviluppo tra Varie Parti del Sistema Nervoso." *Commentationes, Pontificia Academia Scientiarum*, vol. 8 (1944), pp. 527–568.

4. Viktor Hamburger, 1949 (cat. no. 153).

5. Rita Levi-Montalcini, 1949 (cat. no. 154).

6. Elmer Bueker. "Implantation of Tumors in the Hind Limb Field of the Embryonic Chick and the Developmental Response of the Lumbosacral Nervous System." *Anatomical Record*, vol. 102, no. 3 (1948), pp. 369–389.

7. Rita Levi-Montalcini and Viktor Hamburger. "Selective Growth Stimulating Effects of Mouse Sarcoma on the Sensory and Sympathetic Nervous System of the Chick Embryo." *Journal of Experimental Zoology*, vol. 116, no. 2 (1951), pp. 321–361.

8. Stanley Cohen, 1954 (cat. no. 156).

9. Nobel Prize award presentation speech. http://www.nobelprize.org/nobel_prizes/medicine/laureates/1986/presentation-speech.html (accessed January 1, 2013).

## REFERENCES

Hitchcook, Susan Tyler. *Rita Levi-Montalcini: Nobel Prize Winner*. Philadelphia: Chelsea House Publishers, 2005.

Levi-Montalcini, Rita. *In Praise of Imperfection: My Life and Work* [*Elogio dell'imperfezione*]. New York: Basic Books, 1988.

McGrayne, Sharon Bertsch. *Nobel Prize Women in Science: Their Lives, Struggles and Momentous Discoveries*. New York: Birch Lane Press, 1993, pp. 201–224.

152. Rita Levi-Montalcini, cell biologist and 1986 Nobel Laureate, in her laboratory at Washington University, St. Louis, ca.1963. Photograph. (Courtesy, The Bernard Becker Medical Library Digital Collection, Washington University, St. Louis.)

153. Viktor Hamburger and Rita Levi-Montalcini. "Proliferation, Differentiation and Degeneration in the Spinal Ganglia of the Chick Embryo under Normal and Experimental Conditions." *Journal of Experimental Zoology*, vol. 111, no. 3, pp. 457–501 (1949). Bound volume.

In 1944, Levi-Montalcini published her discovery of developmental neural degeneration, based on observing that excision of an embryonic chicken limb resulted in reduced neural size and number in the excised area. Viktor Hamburger had failed to recognize the degenerative process because he had focused on a single developmental end point while she had sampled her specimens over time. This collaborative article demonstrates the correctness of her conclusion. Open to pages 500–501: Plate 1, Fig. 8 shows the abundance of neural material in the side of the embryonic chick with intact wing, in contrast to Fig. 9, with greatly reduced neural material on the ablated side.

154. Rita Levi-Montalcini. "The Development of the Acoustico-vestibular Centers in the Chick Embryo in the Absence of the Afferent Root Fibers and of Descending Fiber Tracts." *Journal of Comparative Neurology*, vol. 91, no. 2, pp. 209–241 (1949). Bound volume. (Courtesy, The New York Academy of Medicine Library.)

Levi-Montalcini demonstrates here that when an embryonic ear is extirpated, nerve cells targeted for that area will die or be greatly reduced in number. She had begun her great scientific career by showing this effect in the motor system, e.g., with the extirpation of a chick wing (see cat. no. 153), and by experimenting now with the effect of extirpation of the embryonic ear, she has generalized her discovery to the sensory system. Open to pages 212–213: Figs. 1 and 2 show the progressive decrease of sensory cells caused by the removal of the embryonic ear on the left side.

155. Rita Levi-Montalcini, Hertha Meyer, and Viktor Hamburger. "In Vitro Experiments on the Effects of Mouse Sarcomas 180 and 37 on the Spinal and Sympathetic Ganglia of the Chick Embryo." *Cancer Research*, vol. 14, no. 1, pp. 49–57 (January 1954). Offprint.

Work with a mouse tumor, sarcoma 180, led Levi-Montalcini to hypothesize a "growth factor" secreted by the tumor that stimulated neural growth. To define the characteristics of this somewhat mysterious substance, she and her colleagues maintained a separation between the neurons and the tumor, and observed that the tumor stimulated prolific neural growth without direct contact, providing indication of the effect of "growth factor" through diffusion. Open to Figs. 13 through 18: Figs. 13 and 15 show that at a distance from the tumor, the neural growth is as super-stimulated as when, Figs. 14 and 16, the tumor touches the neural area.

156. Stanley Cohen, Rita Levi-Montalcini, and Viktor Hamburger. "A Nerve Growth-stimulating Factor Isolated from Sarcoma AS 37 and 180." *Proceedings of the National Academy Sciences USA,* vol. 40, no. 10, pp. 1014–1018 (1954). Offprint. [SEE FIG. 29]

After discovering that "growth factor" could act without direct contact with the tumor (cat. no. 155), the pressing problem became to define that substance causing the extraordinary neural stimulation. This article reports their extraction of the "growth factor" from its tumor source by creating tumor cell-free homogenates, that is, destroying the tumor cells and extracting the liquid substance that stimulated neural growth. Nerve growth factor was shown to be an intracellular cellular substance that did not depend upon the integrity of the sarcoma cells. Open to pages 1017–1018: Fig. 6 shows nerve cells with stimulated growth in the presence of the tumor. The key is Fig. 8, which shows the nerve growth stimulated with the tumor cell-free extract. Numbers 5 and 7 are controls.

157. Stanley Cohen and Rita Levi-Montalcini. "Purification and Properties of a Nerve Growth-promoting Factor Isolated from Mouse Sarcoma 180." *Cancer Research*, vol. 17, no. 1, pp. 15–20 (January 1957). Offprint.

After hypothesizing the existence of "growth factor" and unveiling step-by-step its characteristics (cat. nos. 155 and 156), in a brief three years Cohen and Levi-Montalcini had purified the substance and determined that it had to be a protein or bound to a protein, and that it needed to be continuously present in the cell cultures to be effective. This was the culmination of their work on nerve growth factor, for which they won the Nobel Prize. Open to Figs. 7–9. Figs. 8 and 9 show neural growth stimulated by their purified material. No stimulated neural growth is present in the control, Fig. 7.

158. Rita Levi-Montalcini. *Elogio dell'imperfezione*. Milan: Garzanti, 1987. First edition with dust jacket.

Levi-Montalcini was a prolific author of books outside of her scientific field. This autobiography, however, is the only one that has been translated into English, as *In Praise of Imperfection: My Life and Work* (Reference 3). In writing about the adverse conditions she lived through during World War II, the years of her first great embryological discoveries, in discussing the progressive uncovering of nerve growth factor, and other challenges met and people known, she reveals a side of herself that suggests uncertainty and a sense of fallibility, in contrast to the clarity and decisiveness that characterized her manner of functioning in science, organizational work and political activity.

# GERTY THERESA RADNITZ CORI  1896–1957

BIOGRAPHY

Gerty Theresa Radnitz Cori was born to a distinguished Jewish family in Prague, part of an intellectual circle that included Franz Kafka. Her father, a chemist, managed sugar refineries. After home schooling, Gerty attended a girls' lyceum and then, because of her interest in science, attended the Realgymnasium at Tetschen, graduating in 1914. Encouraged by her uncle, a professor of pediatrics at the University of Prague, she decided to study medicine. Women could be admitted to the University's medical school but needed proficiency in Latin, mathematics, and chemistry or physics, subjects not readily offered to girls. Mastering these with a tutor, she passed the entrance examinations and was admitted to the German branch of Carl Ferdinand University of Prague, graduating with a medical doctor's degree in 1920. In medical school she came to recognize her true vocation: biochemistry. There too, she met another medical student who was to become her life partner – in science and in marriage – Carl Ferdinand Cori, a Catholic from Prague, son of the director of the Marine Biological Station in Trieste.

After WWI, while still medical students, Gerty and Carl, realizing that their interest was research, collaborated on studies of components of blood.[1] In 1920, a banner year for the Coris, they graduated, published the results of their first research, married, and moved to Vienna. There Carl worked in the University's clinic and at the Pharmacology Department of Graz University, while Gerty, working at the Karolinen Children's Hospital, published several papers concerning congenital thyroid deficiency, "cretinism." Although she converted from Judaism to Catholicism so as not hinder Carl's career, and they married within the Catholic Church, they soon realized that her Jewish birth would threaten both their careers. Furthermore, they specifically sought research positions. In 1922 Carl was hired as a biochemist at the New York State Institute for the Study of Malignant Diseases (now Roswell Park Cancer Institute) in Buffalo, and Gerty soon followed as an assistant pathologist. There they worked together for nine years (although the Institute discouraged their collaboration).

After two years during which Gerty studied the effect of x-rays on skin, perhaps with fatal results, they turned to study glucose metabolism.[2] Together they produced fifty scientific papers, placing first the name of whichever had done the major research, and in addition, Gerty published eleven single-authored papers. Their meticulous quantitative studies of the energy metabolism of muscle led to "The Cori Cycle," the explanation of the way the body transforms the food it ingests into energy, which they proposed in 1929,[3] and for which they were ultimately awarded the Nobel Prize.

Although Gerty developed many techniques and carried out studies enabling their discovery, Carl had offers for faculty appointments, turned down because they did not include a position for Gerty. In 1928, the Coris became naturalized United States citizens. Then in 1931, after publishing their work on carbohydrate metabolism, they left Roswell Park for Washington University of St. Louis School of Medicine that, offering Carl chairmanship of the Pharmacology Department, included a position for Gerty as a research assistant (at one-fifth Carl's salary). Here Gerty furthered her investigations of glucose metabolism, and was promoted to research associate professor of biochemistry in 1943. Not until 1947, a year after Carl became chairman of the new Biochemistry Department – and the year Gerty shared the Nobel Prize – did she, the first American woman to win the Nobel Prize and the first woman to win the prize in Physiology or Medicine, become a full professor with tenure and appropriate salary. Gerty, with Carl and Bernardo Alberto Houssay of Argentina, shared the Prize, the Coris for their discoveries concerning glycogen and glucose metabolism, and in particular their synthesis of glycogen.

The Prize Committee defined their great contributions:

> Your magnificent work has now elucidated in great detail the extremely complicated enzymatic mechanism involved in the reversible reactions between glucose and glycogen. Your synthesis of glycogen in the test tube is beyond doubt one of the most brilliant achievements in modern biochemistry.[4]

Gerty went on to bring together her glycogen studies with her initial medical interest in children, studying the enzyme defects in congenital glycogen storage diseases. She discovered four different enzyme deficits that cause different forms of these diseases, which result in muscle weakness, retarded growth, lowered blood sugar and enlarged liver.[5]

In 1947, just before leaving for Stockholm, she was diagnosed with agnogenic myeloid dysplasia, obliteration of blood forming bone marrow cells, perhaps resulting from extensive x-ray exposure during her early studies of x-radiation on skin. The condition is similar to Madame Curie's affliction, both medical martyrs. For ten years Gerty carried out cutting edge science, while receiving blood transfusions and struggling against pain until her death from kidney failure in 1957. She said in 1950, while battling illness, "I came to this country in 1922 and owe it the greatest debt of gratitude for having treated me and my husband with fine generosity, giving us wonderful opportunities for research work, security, and a happy life."[6]

## SIGNIFICANT CONTRIBUTIONS

Carl Cori said: "Our efforts have been largely complementary, and one without the other would not have gone so far. . ."[7] Understanding of that most fundamental process of life, the body's conversion of food into energy, is based upon Gerty Cori's participation in the discovery of the metabolism of carbohydrates, "The Cori Cycle," and the discovery and isolation of the enzymes that enable that process. Standing the test of time, the Cori Cycle remains to this day the explanation of metabolism.

Gerty Cori was the first to show that a defect in an enzyme caused a human genetic disease. Her biochemical analyses of the different forms of glycogen storage diseases enabled her to produce a classification of these diseases on a biochemical level. Six Nobel Laureates received training in the Coris's highly productive laboratory. And among her numerous honors . . . the Cori Crater on the moon and the Cori Crater on Venus are named for her.

RJR AND YK

## ENDNOTES

1. K. Cori and G. Radnitz. "Ueber den Gehalt des menschlichen Blutserums an Komplement und Normalambozeptor für Hammelblutkörperchen." *Zeitschr für Immunitätsforsch und experimentell Therapir*, vol. 29 (1920), pp. 445–462.

2. Gerty Cori. "The Effect of X-rays on the Skin of Vitally Stained White Mice." *Proceedings of the Society for Experimental Biology and Medicine*, vol. 21 (1923), p.123.

3. C. F. Cori and G. T. Cori. "Glycogen Formation in the Liver with d- and l-lactic Acid." *Journal of Biological Chemistry*, vol. 81 (1929), p. 402.

4. Nobel Prize Presentation Speech. http://nobelprize.org/nobel_prizes/medicine/laureates/1947/press.html (accessed January 11, 2013).

5. Cori, 1954 (cat. no. 163).

6. Gerty Theresa Cori. *This I Believe – Gerty T. Cori USA.* CBS Radio Network program hosted by journalist Edward R. Murrow, 1947. http://thisibelieve.org/essay/16457/ (accessed January 11, 2013).

7. Carl Ferdinand Cori. Speech at the Nobel Prize Banquet, Stockholm, Sweden, December 10, 1947. http://www.nobelprize.org/nobel_prizes/medicine/laureates/1947/cori-cf-speech.html?print=1 (accessed January 11, 2013).

## REFERENCES

Cohen, Mildred. "Carl and Gerty Cori: A Personal Recollection." In *Creative Couples in the Sciences*. Eds. Helena M. Pycior, Nancy G. Slack, and Pinna G. Abir-Am. New Brunswick, NJ: Rutgers University Press, 1996, pp. 72–86.

Gerty Cori, Nobel Prize Autobiography, From Nobel Lectures, Physiology or Medicine 1942–1962, Elsevier Publishing Company, Amsterdam, 1964. http://www.nobelprize.org/nobel_prizes/medicine/laureates/1947/cori-gt-bio.html(accessed January 27, 2013).

Larner, Joseph. *Gerty Theresa Cori 1896–1957: A Biographical Memoir. Biographical Memoirs.* Washington, D.C: National Academies Press, 1992, pp.109–135.

McGrayne, Sharon Bertsch. *Nobel Prize Women in Science: Their Lives, Struggles and Momentous Discoveries*. New York: Birch Lane Press, 1993, pp. 93–116.

## ITEMS EXHIBITED

159. Gerty Theresa Cori, biochemist and 1947 Nobel Laureate, working in her laboratory at Washington University, St. Louis. Photograph. (Courtesy, The Bernard Becker Medical Library Digital Collection, Washington University, St. Louis.)

160. A. B. Hegnauer and Gerty T. Cori. "The Influence of Epinephrine on Chemical Changes in Isolated Frog Muscle." *The Journal of Biological Chemistry*, vol. 105, no. 4, pp. 691–703 (July 1934). Offprint.

Using the isolated frog muscle, these studies demonstrate the effect of epinephrine, produced in the adrenalin gland (adrenalin) in increasing the production of biologically active molecules in muscle. Open to pages 696–697, Table II, which shows the increase in lactic acid and hexosephosphate when the muscle is exposed to epinephrine, leading to greater muscular activity.

161. G. T. Cori and C. F. Cori. "The Disappearance of Hexosemonphosphate from Muscle under Aerobic and Anaerobic Con-

8  Disappearance of Hexosephosphate

hydrolysis·value (in N HCl), and the total acid-soluble P were determined in each case. Recovery after stimulation was accompanied by an increase in the directly estimable P, which corresponded closely to the amount of inorganic P liberated by the disappearance of hexosephosphate.

TABLE II

*Disappearance of Hexosephosphate in Frog Muscle with Intact Circulation*

Tetanic stimulation of the lower end of the spinal cord for three 10 second periods with 10 second pauses was applied, except in Experiments 4, 5, and 8, in which sciatic branches of the lower leg muscles were stimulated. The temperature varied between 24–27°. Values are given in mg. per 100 gm. of muscle.

| Experiment No. | 0 min. Hexosephosphate — Hexose | P found | P calcu-lated | Lactic acid | 30 min. Hexosephosphate — Hexose | P found | P calcu-lated | Lactic acid | 60 min. Hexosephosphate — Hexose | P found | P calcu-lated | Lactic acid | 120 min. Hexosephosphate — Hexose | P found | P calcu-lated | Lactic acid |
|---|---|---|---|---|---|---|---|---|---|---|---|---|---|---|---|---|
| 1 | 148 | 28.7 | 25.5 | 212 | 95* | 19.0 | 16.4 | 130 | | | | | | | | |
| 2 | 193 | 32.2 | 33.3 | 89 | 98 | 18.1 | 16.9 | 66 | | | | | | | | |
| 3 | 162 | 27.5 | 27.9 | 109 | 105 | 18.9 | 18.1 | 46 | | | | | | | | |
| 4 | 207 | 37.9 | 35.7 | 92 | 108 | 18.7 | 18.6 | 19 | | | | | | | | |
| 5 | 168 | 27.8 | 29.0 | 95 | 110 | 18.6 | 19.0 | 22· | | | | | | | | |
| 6† | 130 | 21.0 | 22.4 | 180 | 104 | 18.5 | 17.9 | 114 | | | | | | | | |
| 7† | 93 | 15.8 | 16.0 | | 74 | 11.9 | 12.7 | | | | | | | | | |
| 8 | | | | | 107 | 19.6 | 18.4 | 25 | 93 | 16.3 | 16.0 | 22 | | | | |
| 9 | | | | | 120 | 21.3 | 21.4 | 79 | 106 | 19.9 | 18.3 | 65 | | | | |
| 10 | | | | | | | | | 105 | 20.7 | 18.1 | 79 | 77 | 14.7 | 13.3 | 45 |
| 11 | | | | | | | | | 81 | 13.6 | 14.0 | 64 | 63 | 10.9 | 10.9 | 35 |
| 12 | | | | | | | | | | | | | 45 | 8.3 | 7.8 | 18 |

\* 15 minutes after stimulation.
† Single shocks at a rate of 54 per minute for 15 minutes.

The rate of aerobic disappearance of hexosephosphate does not seem to be influenced by the lactic acid concentration present in muscle, at least within the range of variations encountered in these experiments. After stimulation of both hind limbs through the spinal cord (Experiments 1 to 3) the lactic acid content of

Fig. 30. Table II from G. T. Cori and C. F. Cori. "The Disappearance of Hexosemonphosphate from Muscle under Aerobic and Anaerobic Conditions," *The Journal of Biological Chemistry*, vol. 107, no. 1, pp. 5–12 (October 1934) shows the results of stimulation of frog muscle under aerobic conditions. [CAT. 161]

ditions." *The Journal of Biological Chemistry*, vol. 107, no. 1, pp. 5–12 (October 1934). Offprint. [SEE FIG. 30]

This comparative study demonstrates that after stimulation to a frog muscle by electric shock, hexosemonphosphate, a product of muscle contraction, disappears more quickly in a muscle exposed to oxygen through blood circulation than in a muscle in an anaerobic context. This is one of many studies through which the Coris discovered the essential metabolic process, the Cori Cycle, for which they were awarded the Nobel Prize. Open to pages 8–9, Table II, showing the results of stimulation under aerobic conditions.

162. G. T. Cori, S. P. Colowick, and C. F. Cori. "The Action of Nucleotides in the Disruptive Phosphorylation of Glycogen." *The Journal of Biological Chemistry*, vol. 123, no. 2, pp. 381–389 (1938). Offprint.

This article exemplifies the exquisite refinement of studies that were essential to reach a comprehensive understanding of glycogen metabolism. Open to pages 384–385, Figs. 1 and 2, which plot the effects of substances that inhibit the metabolism of glycogen in the muscle; the higher the curve, the greater the inhibition.

163. G. T. Cori. "Glycogen Structure and Enzyme Deficiencies in Glycogen Storage Disease." *The Harvey Lectures,* vol. 48, pp. 145–171. New York: Academic Press, 1954. Offprint.

Having discovered the Cori Cycle, and been awarded the Nobel Prize, Gerty Cori, turning her focus to a new challenge, became the first to demonstrate the biochemical basis of a genetic disease. Her March 19, 1953 lecture summarizes her work concerning glycogen storage diseases, which in most patients cause severe liver pathology. Open to pages 162–163, Table 5 shows the abnormally low glucose activity in affected patients. Fig. 5 is a microscopic photograph showing the abnormality of the cells in a patient's liver.

# GERTRUDE BELLE ELION  1918–1999

## BIOGRAPHY

Gertrude Belle Elion was born in New York City on January 23, 1918. Her emigrant father, like her mother, came from a line of scholars and rabbis, and worked as a dentist and stockbroker until the crash of 1929 forced the family's move from Manhattan to the Bronx.

Graduating in 1933 from the girls' Walton High School in the Bronx, and earning membership in the National Honor Society, Arista, Elion continued her education at Hunter College for women. Elected to Phi Beta Kappa, and graduating at nineteen with a B.A. in chemistry, she was rejected from fifteen graduate chemistry departments, very possibly because she was a woman. As one university told her, "You're qualified. But we've never had a woman in the laboratory before and we think it would be a distracting influence."[1]

She entered secretarial school while working part-time teaching chemistry to nursing students at New York Hospital School of Nursing for $200. Soon, though, Denver Chemical Company in New York City offered her a position, at first unsalaried, but later raised to $20 a week. Living at home for eighteen months, she saved $450, enough to pay for one year of graduate study, and finally obtained admission to New York University's chemistry program, earning her master's degree in 1941, the only woman in her class. While a graduate student, she worked as a receptionist, took education classes, and became a substitute teacher.

World War II, with men away, improved women's employment opportunities. Elion was hired to test food products for A&P stores where she learned much about instrumentation and quality control and, in 1944, she went to work at Johnson & Johnson research laboratories; when her unit closed, she was offered another position testing the tensile strength of surgical sutures, but she was looking to make a more substantial contribution.

Her dentist father, receiving a sample of Empirin from Burroughs Wellcome Company in Tuckahoe, New York, suggested she apply there for a research position. There was an opening: they hired her. Her supervisor and coworker was the biochemist George Hitchings, whose work seeking antagonists to nucleic acid derivatives excited her and broadened her view of possibilities for cancer research. She remained in this laboratory for the rest of her career, becoming head of the

Department of Experimental Therapy in 1967; here she made her world famous, life saving discoveries in chemotherapeutic agents against cancer and viruses.

While working at research, Elion also pursued a doctorate at Brooklyn Polytechnic Institute but the institution denied her permission to continue graduate studies part-time. Choosing to continue investigations into purines and purine analogs as chemotherapeutic agents, she set aside the doctorate. In 1969 George Mandell of Washington University in St. Louis telephoned her: "Look, the kind of work you're doing, you've long since passed what a doctorate would have meant. But we've got to make an honest woman of you. We'll give you a doctorate, so we can call you 'doctor' legitimately," the first of her many honorary doctorates – including one from Brooklyn Polytechnic Institute.[2]

In 1988, she was awarded the Nobel Prize in Medicine, shared with colleagues James Black and George Hitchings. Her Nobel was unique in that she had no Ph.D. degree, and was a pharmaceutical firm employee – not a "regular academic." In commenting on her years grappling with frustration and discrimination, Elion said, "The Nobel Prize was icing on the cake. The thrill of seeing people get well who might otherwise have died of disease. . . cannot be described in words."[3]

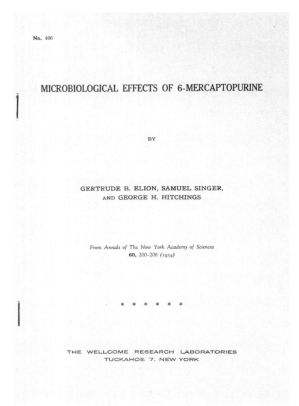

Fig. 31. Cover page of offprint: Gertrude B. Elion, Samuel Singer, and George H. Hitchings. "Microbiological Effects of 6-mercaptopurine." *Annals of the New York Academy of Sciences*, vol. 60, no. 2, pp. 200–206 (1954), in which it is demonstrated that 6-mercaptopurine interferes with the multiplication of cells, bringing about remission of childhood leukemia, the first chemotherapeutic treatment clinically effective against a cancer. [CAT. 165]

## SIGNIFICANT CONTRIBUTIONS

In the 1950s, Elion participated in developing drugs that created remission in childhood leukemia, the first chemotherapeutic agents effective against cancer. Since the effect of these compounds, including 6-mercaptopurine (6-MP) which she had designed against leukemia, was not long lasting, she created drug combinations that included 6-MP and that cured most childhood leukemia, the first chemotherapeutic cure developed against cancer.[4,5]

There were, at the time, no medicines or chemicals to counter viral illness. Elion investigated what allows viruses to live and multiply, and how they also protect themselves from death. She and her colleagues – going beyond the old way of serially trying compounds off the shelf – rationally created substances effective in mitigating or eliminating the virus's disease-causing properties, whether by altering its metabolism or by killing it. She was instrumental in developing Acyclovir,[6,7,8] turning the tables on the view that "nothing could stop a virus." The idea that viral infections could be cured met with intense skepticism and resistance, until finally, with her presentation of thirteen posters at the Atlanta Interscience Conference on Antimicrobial Agents and Chemotherapy in 1978, the world recognized what she had achieved.[9] Acyclovir is effective against many viral diseases, including herpes, and is the basis for developing AZT for the treatment of AIDS.

She also synthesized azathiopurine (trade name Imuran), based upon 6-MP, that prevents organ transplantation rejection,[10] further developed by Robert Schwartz in rabbits,[11] and applied to the first transplants of kidneys in unrelated people by Joseph E Murray,[12] for which Murray received the Nobel Prize in 1990. Today Imuran is a mainstay of transplantation surgery. Allopurinol, also synthesized by Elion, is now used worldwide for the treatment of the debilitating disease gout.[13]

Elion's knowledge-based system of designing drugs against disease established the rationale for all subsequent drug development. Today almost every effective drug intervention is based on Elion's concept of understanding cellular mechanisms and, with molecular biologists and biochemists, developing drugs to interfere with the functioning of pathological cells.

Among appreciative letters Elion kept in her desk that gave her further stimulus for her work, one reads:

Dear Ms. Elion:
I open my newspaper this morning and through many tears read of your great honor, Nobel Prize. My daughter Tiffany was stricken with herpes encephalitis in Septem-

ber 1987, a neurologist, said the only help for hope for her was possibly the drug acyclovir.

I thank the Lord, so many times that he blessed you with determination, stamina, love, in patience to work all the long hours, days, months, and years it takes to invent a new drug. Tiffany is a senior in high school this year and doing great. May the Lord bless you beyond your wildest dreams.

Tiffany's mother.[14]

RJR AND YK

## ENDNOTES

1. Sharon Bertsch McGrayne. "Damn the Torpedoes. Full Speed Ahead!" *Science*, vol. 296, no. 5569 (2002), pp. 851–852.

2. McGrayne, p. 298, 1993.

3. McGrayne, 2002.

4. George H. Hitchings, Gertrude B. Elion, E. A. Falco, R. B. Russell, and H. van der Werff. "Studies on Analogs of Purines and Pyrimidines." *Annals of the New York Academy of Sciences,* vol. 52, no. 8 (1950), pp. 1318–1335.

5. Gertrude B. Elion, Samuel Singer and George H. Hitchings. "Microbiological Effects of 6-mercaptopurine," 1954 (cat. no. 165).

6. Gertrude B. Elion, Janet L. Rideout, Paulo de Miranda, Peter Collins, and D. J. Bauer, 1975 (cat. no. 167).

7. Gertrude B. Elion, Phillip A. Furman, James A. Fyfe, Paulo de Miranda, Lilia Beauchamp, and Howard J. Schaeffer. "Selectivity of Action of an Antiherpetic Agent, 9-(2-hydroxyethoxymethyl) guanine." *Proceedings of the National Academy of Sciences USA*, vol. 74, no. 12 (1977), pp. 5716–5720.

8. Hans J. Schaeffer, Lilia de M. P. Beauchamp, Gertrude B. Elion, D. J. Bauer, and Peter Collins. "9-(2-hydroxyethoxymethyl) Guanine Activity against Viruses of the Herpes Group." *Nature*, vol. 272, no. 5654 (1978), pp. 583–585.

9. Personal communication. Sharon Bertsch McGrayne, May 12, 2012.

10. Gertrude B. Elion. "Pharmacologic and Physical Agents. Immunosuppressive Agents." *Transplant Proceedings*, vol. 9, no. 1 (1977), pp. 975–979.

11. R. Schwartz, J. K. Stack, and W. Dameshek. "Effect of 6-mercaptopurine on Antibody Production." *Proceedings of the Society for Experimental Biology and Medicine*, vol. 99, no. 1 (1958), pp.164–167.

12. Joseph E. Murray, John P. Merrill, Gustave J. Dammin, James B. Dealy Jr., George W. Alexander, and J. Hartwell Harrison. "Kidney Transplantation in Modified Recipients." *Annals of Surgery*, vol. 156, pp. 337–355.

13. Gertrude B. Elion. "Enzymatic and Metabolic Studies with Allopurinol." *Annals of the Rheumatic Diseases*, vol. 25, Suppl. 6 (1966), pp. 608–614.

14. Dora Shaw letter, 1988 (cat. no. 169).

REFERENCES

Gertrude Elion (1918–1999). American Chemical Society http://portal.acs.org/portal/acs/corg/content?_nfpb=true&_pageLabel=PP_ARTICLEMAIN&node_id=124&content_id=CNBP_026830&use_sec=true&sec_url_var=region1&__uuid=36a0698b-0b68-4f8b-86c1-68e1346571c5 (accessed January 6, 2013).

"Gertrude B. Elion – Autobiography." Nobelprize.org. From Les Prix Nobel. The Nobel Prizes 1988. Ed. Tore Frängsmyr. Stockholm: [Nobel Foundation] http://www.nobelprize.org/nobel_prizes/medicine/laureates/1988/elion.html (accessed January 7, 2013).

Sharon Bertsch McGrayne. *Nobel Prize Women in Science: Their Lives, Struggles, and Momentous Discoveries.* New York: Birch Lane Press, 1993, pp. 280–303.

"Physiology or Medicine 1988 – Press Release." http://nobelprize.org/nobel_prizes/medicine/laureates/1988/press.http (accessed January 12, 2013).

ITEMS EXHIBITED

164. Gertrude Elion, biochemist and 1988 Nobel Laureate, in her laboratory at Burroughs Wellcome Co. Photograph. (Courtesy, *Britannica Online*.)

165. Gertrude B. Elion, Samuel Singer, and George H. Hitchings. "Microbiological Effects of 6-mercaptopurine." *Annals of the New York Academy of Sciences*, vol. 60, no. 2, pp. 200–206, New York, 1954. Offprint. [SEE FIG. 31]

Elion designed 6-mercaptopurine (6-MP), a chemotherapeutic treatment which brought about remission in childhood leukemia, the first effective agent developed against a cancer. The drug she designed, 6-Thioguanine, also investigated in this study, in combination with 6-MP and other drugs *cured* most childhood leukemia, the first chemotherapeutic cure ever developed against a cancer. Open to pages 204–205: Table 2 shows that, using bacteria as an early model, 6-MP, designed as a potential drug to treat leukemia, decreases the number of bacteria by 85%.

166. Gertrude B. Elion. "Drugs in the Treatment of Hyperuricemia." *Advances in Nephrology,* vol. 3 (1974), pp. 51–57. Offprint.

Gout is usually caused by abnormal purine metabolism that leads to an intensely painful buildup of uric acid in vulnerable joints. Only pain palliatives were available at the time, but no medication to inhibit the disease process. Elion had invented the drug allopurinol to improve the effectiveness of 6-MP in treating leukemia, but the combination didn't work, and so allopurinol was set aside until, as this article summarizes, Elion showed its effectiveness in interfering with the buildup of uric acid: to this day it is a first line medication against gout.

167. Gertrude B. Elion, et al. "Biological Activities of some Purine Arabinosides." *Annals of the New York Academy of Sciences*, vol. 255, pp. 468–480 (1975). Offprint.

This article takes up Elion's game-changing development of antiviral compounds. The drugs administered enabled almost all of the treated mice (closed circles in the illustration) to survive a dose of viral meningitis, delivered directly to the brain, 1000 times greater than what would be needed to kill 50% of the mice not treated with the antiviral compounds. Open to pages 470–471, Figs. 3 and 4. Fig. 3 shows that, in the mouse model, antivirals greatly increased survival from viral meningitis.

168. Gertrude B. Elion. The Purine Path to Chemotherapy – Nobel Lecture. *Bioscience Reports*, vol. 9, no. 5, pp. 509–529 (1989). Offprint.

Elion concluded her Nobel Prize Lecture delivered December 8, 1988:

*In my attempt to cover 40 years of research on purines and purine analogs, I have been able to give only a bird's eye view. However, I hope that I have successfully conveyed our philosophy that chemotherapeutic agents are not only ends in themselves, but also serve as tools for unlocking doors and probing Nature's mysteries. This approach has served us well and has led into many new areas of medical research. Selectivity remains our aim and understanding its basis our guide to the future.*

169. Dora Shaw (Tiffany's mother), personal letter of thanks to Gertrude B. Elion and George H. Hitchings, October 9, 1988. (Courtesy, Dr. Jon Elion.)

Dr. Jon Elion, Gertrude Elion's nephew, wrote in personal correspondence: "Trudy had always said that the letters from patients were more important to her than the Nobel Prize itself (or any other recognition)." Dr. Elion informed us that he had found in a box among saved treasures two things: "First, the actual Nobel citation, the one handed to her during the ceremonies by the King. The other was a manila folder simply labeled "Patients."

# ROSALYN SUSSMAN YALOW 1921–2011

## BIOGRAPHY

Rosalyn Yalow was born in the Bronx to Simon Sussman, a wholesaler of packaging materials, and Clara Zipper, neither of whom had a high school education, but both of whom held literacy in the highest esteem. Rosalyn was reading before kindergarten and went weekly with her brother to borrow books from the public library. She, like Gertrude Elion before her, attended the girls' Walton High School in the Bronx, and was already deeply involved in mathematics when a teacher excited her interest in chemistry. She then, as Elion had, enrolled in Hunter College,

New York City's free college for women. She has said that two events ignited her interest in physics: reading Eve Curie's biography of her mother, Marie Curie and, in her junior year, 1939, hearing Enrico Fermi lecture on nuclear fission. She was Hunter College's first physics major, graduating *magna cum laude* in 1941.

That did not, however, offer access to graduate school. As Purdue University wrote to her Hunter professor, "She is from New York. She is Jewish. She is a woman."[1] The future Nobel Prize laureate, therefore, took a secretarial job and enrolled in business school.

But as World War II opened opportunities for women, Yalow was accepted with a teaching assistantship in the Engineering College of the University of Illinois in 1941, the first woman in that graduate program since 1917, when World War I had eased the possibility of graduate study for women. There she met Aaron Yalow, a physics graduate student, and they married in 1943. As the only woman in a class of 400, she felt pressure to prove herself: an A- in a lab course led the Physics Department's chairman to conclude " . . . women do not do well at lab work," but she remained, she said, " . . . a stubborn, determined graduate student,"[2] and in 1945 received her Ph.D. in nuclear physics.

She returned to New York as a research assistant and the sole woman engineer for the Federal Telecommunications Laboratory, but when her research group left New York, she returned to Hunter to teach physics to veterans. She also volunteered in a medical lab at Columbia University where she received some training in the new field of medical uses of radioisotopes. This was a stroke of luck: the Veterans Administration Hospitals, wanting to establish radiotherapy services, hired her in 1947 as a part-time consultant to their Bronx hospital. By 1950, she was working full time and had begun her fruitful collaboration with Solomon A. Berson, an internist at the VA, which lasted until his death in 1972.

Yalow and Berson, using radioisotopes, began studying blood volume, iodine metabolism, and thyroid disease, which led them to study the hormone insulin. Here began their discoveries through which they solved pressing issues of medical diagnosis and treatment.

Yalow and Berson had two patient groups with insulin deficiency: those who had never received insulin and those who had (diabetics and schizophrenics who had insulin shock therapy). They determined that the levels of radioactive insulin disappeared more slowly in patients with previous insulin experience than in those new to insulin,[3,4] observations inconsistent with the contemporary dogma that abnormally rapid degradation of insulin by the liver caused insulin deficiency. They reasoned that the retardation of the hepatic breakdown of insulin was caused by the presence of an insulin antibody developed by the immune system in response to the earlier insulin experience, and so was primed to bind to newly introduced insulin molecules. They realized also that, in contrast to methods requiring large quantities of blood to perform an assay, radioisotopes allowed measurements to be made with a drop of blood, far more feasible and far less costly.

Yet, the resistance to their new ideas was so great that it took three years before they succeeded in publishing their antibody observations – and then only after they agreed to eliminate the controversial world "antibody" from the title of their article!

Their insulin work led to their next revelation: their technique for detecting antibodies could be expanded to measure many essential and medically critical bodily substances. The discovery of radioimmunoassay (RIA) revolutionized diagnostic medicine.

Rosalyn Yalow, in 1976, was the first woman to receive the Lasker Award in basic medical research and in 1977 the second American woman – the first was Gerty Cori – awarded the Nobel Prize in Physiology or Medicine. She felt deeply the irony that Dr. Berson, who died in 1972, could not share the Nobel Prize, which cannot be awarded posthumously, and paid gracious tribute to him in her Nobel address:

> From 1950 until his untimely death in 1972, Dr. Solomon Berson was joined with me in this scientific adventure and together we gave birth to and nurtured through its infancy radioimmunoassay, a powerful tool for determination of virtually any substance of biologic interest. Would that he were here to share this moment.[5]

Yalow developed other applications for RIA and her VA laboratory became the world wide training center. She was appointed Chair of the new Clinical Science Department at Montefiore Medical Center in 1980, the first woman to head a department at that institution.[6]

It is important, considering the path of some recent scientific discoveries, that Yalow and Berson *never patented their discoveries*:

> In my day, scientists didn't patent things. You did it for people. Unfortunately, now is not the way life was. What would we have done with the money except poured it into research? . . . If I had $5 billion a year for research, it would be necessary for me to supervise 100 scientists. It would be impossible for me to talk to each of them every day . . . I'm psychologically adjusted to 'mom and pop' science.[7]

## SIGNIFICANT CONTRIBUTIONS

Radioimmunoassay, through which minute quantities of biological substances – antibodies, antigens, hormones, vitamins and other substances – can be detected, opened new areas of biological research, and has brought about the identification, cure and care of heretofore devastating diseases. One example: the use of RIA to diagnosis hypothyroidism in newborns through a drop of blood has saved countless thousands of infants from severe metal retardation.

RJR AND YK

## ENDNOTES

1. McGrayne, p. 338.

2. "Rosalyn Yalow – Banquet speech". The Nobel Prize in Physiology or Medicine 1977 http://www.nobelprize.org/nobel_prizes/medicine/laureates/1977/yalow-speech.html (accessed March 1, 2013).

3. Solomon A. Berson, Rosalyn S. Yalow, A. Bauman, M. A. Rothschild, and K. Newerly (cat. no. 171).

4. Rosalyn S. Yalow and Solomon A. Berson (cat. no. 172).

5. Yalow, Nobel Lecture.

6. http://www.ncbi.nlm.nih.gov/pubmed (accessed January 4, 2013).

7. McGrayne, p. 349.

## REFERENCES

McGrayne, Sharon Bertsch, *Nobel Prize Women in Science: Their Lives, Struggles and Momentous Discoveries*. New York: Birch Lane Press, 1993, pp. 333–355.

Rall, J. E. "Solomon A. Berson: 1918–1972." http://www.nasonline.org/publications/biographical-memoirs/memoir-pdfs/berson-solomon-a.pdf (accessed January 4, 2013).

"Rosalyn Yalow – Autobiography". http://www.nobelprize.org/nobel_prizes/medicine/laureates/1977/yalow.html (accessed March 1, 2013).

Stone, Elizabeth, "A Mme. Curie from the Bronx," *New York Times*, April 9, 1978.

Straus, Eugene. *Rosalyn Yalow Nobel Laureate: Her Life and Work in Medicine*. New York and London: Plenum Press, 1998.

## ITEMS EXHIBITED

170. Rosalyn Sussman Yalow, biochemist and 1977 Nobel Laureate, preparing a radio-iodine mixture used in thyroid diagnostic procedures. Photograph. (Courtesy, The Radioisotope Unit, Veterans Administration Hospital, Bronx, New York.)

171. Solomon A. Berson, et al. "Insulin-I$^{131}$ Metabolism in Human Subjects: Demonstration of Insulin Binding Globulin in the Circulation of Insulin Treated Subjects."

*The Journal of Clinical Investigation*, vol. 35, no. 2, pp. 170–190 (1956). Bound volume.

Insulin antibodies were the first great discovery using radioimmunoassay (RIA). In insulin-deficient patients who were administered radioactive insulin, the insulin disappeared faster in those physiologically naïve to insulin than in those who had received it previously. This revealed the primed immune system's antibody response. *Note what's missing from the article's title*: resistance to the new ideas was so great that it took three years before they succeeded in publishing their antibody observations – and then only after they agreed to eliminate the offending world "antibody" from the title! Open to Table II, p. 185, which tabulates the described difference.

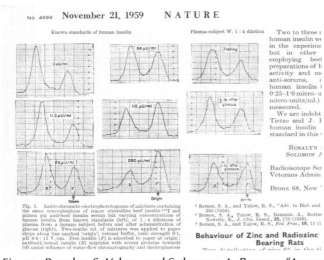

Fig. 32. Rosalyn S. Yalow and Solomon A. Berson. "Assay of Plasma Insulin in Human Subjects by Immunological Methods." *Nature*, vol. 184, no. 4699, pp. 1648–1649 (November 21, 1959). [CAT. 172]

172. Rosalyn S. Yalow and Solomon A. Berson. "Assay of Plasma Insulin in Human Subjects by Immunological Methods." *Nature*, vol. 184, no. 4699, pp. 1648–1649 (November 21, 1959). Bound volume. [SEE FIG. 32]

This brief note in *Nature* demonstrates the exquisite sensitivity of radioimmunoassay: Yalow and Berson were able to detect two to three micro units of human insulin, heretofore undetectable. In contrast to former methods requiring large quantities of blood, measurements could be made with just a drop of blood, making immunoassay far more feasible and far less costly, allowing for a vast increase in efficiency and effectiveness in medical diagnosis. Open to pages 1648 and 1649, with a full graphical portrayal of the report.

173. Solomon A. Berson (deceased) and Rosalyn S. Yalow, eds. *Methods in Investigation and Diagnostic Endocrinology. Peptide Hormones*. Amsterdam and London: North-Holland Publishing Company, 1973.

This book, published shortly after Berson's death, brings together in thirty chapters all current applications of radioimmunoassay. Although Yalow and Berson struggled to achieve publication of their discovery, seventeen years later, the uses of radioimmunoassay have expanded vastly and it has become the standard worldwide. Open to *Abbreviated contents*, that shows utility in assaying almost every known hormone.

# INDEX